D1536330

NATURE'S MIRACLES

73 (New) Alternatives to Modern Medicine

With Commonsense Tips and Tricks to
Take Charge of Your Health

by *Andy Snyder*

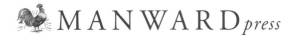

MANWARD *press*

ABOUT MANWARD PRESS

Manward Press is an ultra-unique lifestyle and financial publisher that focuses on just one thing: sharing ideas that lead men to richer, healthier, fuller lives that overflow with freedom. At Manward's core is a belief that men who focus on three scientifically proven principles – Liberty, Know-How and Connections, aka the "Triad" – are happier and more successful.

More information can be found at ManwardPress.com.

© 2019 Manward Press | All Rights Reserved

Manward Press is a financial and lifestyle publisher that does not offer any personal financial or medical advice. The information provided in this book should not be construed as personal medical advice or instruction. No action should be taken based solely on the contents of this book. Readers should consult appropriate health professionals on any matter relating to their health and well-being.

Protected by copyright laws of the United States and international treaties. The information found in this book may only be used pursuant to the membership or subscription agreement and any reproduction, copying or redistribution (electronic or otherwise, including on the world wide web), in whole or in part, is strictly prohibited without the express written permission of Manward Press, 14 West Mount Vernon Place, Baltimore, MD 21201.

What's Inside

Part III: Know-How in Action

Part IV: Recipes for a Healthy Mind

Part V: A Critical Look at Men's Health

Part VI: 21st-Century Illnesses

A Healthy Distrust of the System Is... Healthy

We once had a ram that liked to chase our wife.

Whether the year-old sheep just wanted to put on a show, got overly excited for some hay or was protecting his flock, we're not sure.

It doesn't matter. Rams will be rams.

It's life on our microfarm.

A lot of folks have asked us why we put up with it... why we spend so much time nurturing our crops and critters. The list of answers is as long as our arm. Lifestyle... discipline... a reliable source of food... they could all stand on their own.

But lately, we've added another.

You see, our trust is waning.

Your Life vs. Their Word

Much of our food is produced in a factory – in a process that's not all that different from making a chunk of plastic.

Sure, that cow in your burger may have grown up on a pasture.

But by the time it gets sliced, diced and put in a nice little wrapper at the grocery store, it's been injected with drugs, flash-frozen in a chemical atmosphere and preserved until even a roach won't touch it.

We're told the process is harmless. The government gives us its guarantee.

But – perhaps it's the onset of old age – we're skeptical. And we'd rather be chased by a ram than find the "experts" were wrong.

It's happened before.

And folks are dead because of it.

We've been studying the nation's opioid addiction.

Hundreds of thousands of Americans have needlessly died or become addicted to prescription pills... all because the medical community was wrong.

It promised we were safe... but we weren't.

You see, in January of 1980, *New England Journal of Medicine* published a short 11-line letter from a couple of doctors who had studied opioids – drugs made from the poppy plant. They claimed, "The development of addiction is rare in medical patients with no history of addiction."

A few years later, a similar paper was published. It claimed that "opioid maintenance therapy can be a safe, salutary and more humane alternative" than surgery or lesser treatments.

Those beliefs led to huge changes in the way doctors treated pain. And it changed the way drugs were sold. Many opioids were marketed as safe and addiction-free.

Wow, were they wrong.

The medical community is paying the price. It's now in the midst of one of the largest self-made epidemics in history.

And recent research from the National Safety Council shows this whole crisis is for naught.

Heroin-like drugs are not the best painkillers – at least not for the patient. No, the answer to all that ails you is already in your medicine cabinet.

It turns out, the research shows, "The combination of 200 mg of ibuprofen and 500 mg of acetaminophen is one of the strongest pain reliever combinations available. It is clearly more efficacious than any of the opioids used alone or in combination with acetaminophen."

Of course, it's not the only time the smartest folks in the room were wrong.

When We Got Smoked

Let's not forget the great tobacco mix-up. How many folks died because our docs were once convinced smoking was not only harmless... but good for us?

After all, the ads told us "More doctors smoke Camels than any other cigarette!"

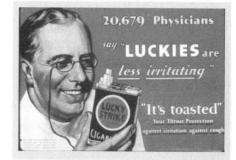

But Lucky Strikes, well, they're great on your throat.

How wrong we were.

It took nearly 30 years for the medical community to fully embrace the dangers of cigarettes.

By then, countless addicts were formed and lives were harmed.

As we let our mind wander, we think of other things that once were accepted as safe but we now know are quite deadly.

Do you remember the fluoroscope? Kids loved taking X-rays of their feet to find the best-fitting shoe. And we didn't hesitate to expose our bodies to their wondrous rays.

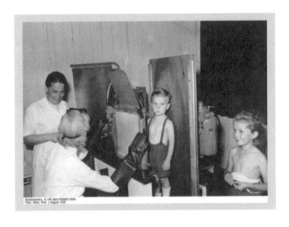

It's crazy now, but in the 1900s, radioactive drinks were popular.

And not long after that, sugar was promoted as a weight-loss aid. "Have a soft drink before your main meal," we were told, or "Snack on some candy an hour before lunch."

Wrong... and wrong.

Passing the Buck

In many cases, the medical community is innocent. It simply doesn't understand the science or, more often, it doesn't have enough time to study the downside.

After all, many of these deadly concoctions take years to kill.

And yet they hit the market quite quickly. (We're already pondering if someday we'll regret what the internet has done to our social skills.)

When it comes to cancer-causing chemicals, our longer life spans play a role, too.

Generations past didn't live long enough to see the downside of their dangerous, cancer-causing habits. But now that the average American can expect to live to nearly 80 years old, that's changed... quickly.

In many other cases, though, there are clearly guilty parties.

That was the case at Purdue Pharma, the company that hid the deadly addictive nature of its opiate OxyContin. Three of its top bosses pleaded guilty, and the company paid a $635 million settlement to Washington.

Meanwhile, innocent folks are still addicted to its pills.

That's why we're careful not to jump to conclusions. It's why we don't trust somebody just because he has a few initials after his name (we do, too, but we sure aren't perfect). And it's why we'd rather do it ourselves than rely on the word of somebody else.

Our farm isn't easy to run. Rams attack. Bees sting. And the hawks love our chickens as much as we do.

But the alternative isn't so grand, either.

A healthy distrust of the system is, well, healthy.

My Mission

My singular goal with everything related to Manward is to take what I've learned from a life of research and lead folks to richer, healthier and more fulfilled lives through our Triad of three scientifically proven principles: Liberty, Know-How and Connections.

I can lead them to increased wealth by diving into the markets and revealing the truth about how to make money in stocks.

I can teach folks a thing or two about using their hands.

I can lead them to better relationships by looking at the many, many things that get in the way.

And – why I've written this book – with a bit of Know-How and the wisdom that comes only with experience, I can give them the tools to take charge of their health.

I've spent countless hours poring over the latest research on the benefits and risks of what goes into our bodies (from both diet and environment)... exploring commonsense wisdom... and debunking quite a few commonly held beliefs about food, diet and health along the way.

Read this book carefully and come back to it often. I beg you.

What's inside may very well save your – or a loved one's – life.

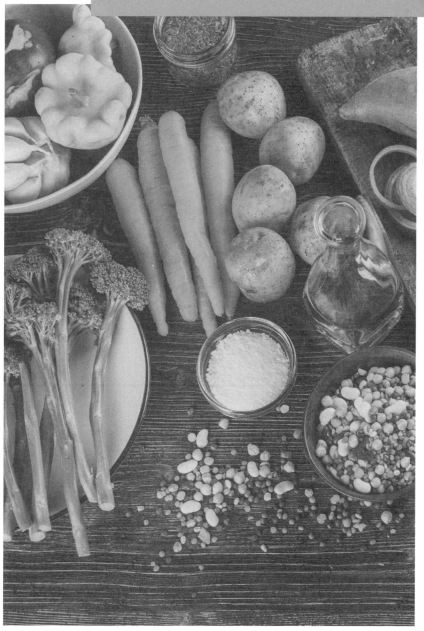

When It Comes to Food, Bigger Isn't Better

Modern agricultural practices are doing far more harm than most folks know.

We're told that genetic engineering won't hurt us... that it leads to bigger crops that can feed the world for less.

Bigger yields? True.

Feed the world? Far from it.

Big Crops, Little Food

Here's the deal. A study from the University of Texas showed definitive proof that modern vegetables aren't what they once were.

A team of scientists looked at 43 crops. They wanted to see whether modern crops contained the same vitamins and nutrients they did in the 1950s.

The news was not good.

Declines for key nutrients, including iron, calcium, protein and others, ranged from 6% to 38%.

With broccoli, for example, a USDA test in 1950 showed 130 mg of calcium. The modern sample researchers poked and prodded, though, showed just 48 mg.

"[Since the 1950s] there have been intensive efforts to breed new varieties that have greater yield or resistance to pests or adaptability to different climates," the study's lead researcher said. "But the dominant effort is for higher yields. Emerging evidence suggests that when you select for yield, crops grow bigger and faster, but they don't necessarily have the ability to make or uptake nutrients at the same, faster rate."

The test shed light on our country's disheartening trend toward quantity over quality.

The researchers in Texas aren't alone. A separate study showed similar results:

- Calcium levels were down 27%.
- Vitamin A was down 21%.
- Vitamin C was down 30%.

And yet another study showed that we'd have to eat eight modern oranges to get the same amount of vitamin A our grandparents would have gotten from eating just one.

Treating Soil Like Dirt

What gives?

It's no surprise that modern farming practices are the culprit.

All we have to do is look out our back windows to see it in action. Our microfarm borders a large commercial farm.

Every year we've lived here... it's been a cornfield.

The cycle is always the same.

The weeds are killed... the corn is planted... the stalks suck up the nutrients... the ears are harvested.

It'll be the same thing next year. Kill the weeds... plant the corn... suck up the nutrients.

Every two years or so, a tractor will visit the field and spread some fertilizer. But no farmer wants to fertilize. It costs money and has some nasty side effects.

Instead, the trend is to grow engineered crops that don't need fertilizer.

Like any good businessmen, farmers want to do more with less.

But the harm these practices have had is undeniable.

Finding Good Food

Our food isn't what it used to be. We pick up an orange, and it lies to us.

Admittedly, we once were skeptics of the organic food trend (we're skeptics of a lot of things). But then we stumbled upon this research. The facts are undeniable.

Organic fruits and vegetables are the best solution.

That's because crops raised without the aid of synthetic chemicals are forced to work harder. They may not be as pretty or as big, but they're a whole lot healthier.

In fact, a study by Dr. Alyson Mitchell showed that organic tomatoes can have as much as 30% more nutrients than conventional ones.

"By avoiding synthetic fertilizers," she said, "organic farmers put more stress on plants, and when plants experience stress, they protect themselves by producing phytochemicals."

There are some tricks we use to find the best and healthiest fruits and vegetables.

First, we look for bright colors. It's typically a sign of a crop with heavy nutrients. We've all seen it... a healthy head of lettuce with deep, rich colors... or a tomato with a crisp, dark red skin.

And we don't always go for the biggest apple in the bunch. Bigger isn't always better in the natural world.

The soil and the plant that depends on it has only so much nutrients (less now than ever). The bigger the crop, the more diluted the healthy vitamins and sugars.

Finally, we look for heirloom varieties. These fruits and vegetables haven't been modified to grow big and fast. (And, not surprisingly, their seeds are currently being stockpiled by governments around the world, but that's another story.) No, they're from a day when industrial farming and high-tech fertilizer and weed killers were still a thing of the future.

They grow slow and small, but they're packed with nutrients.

We're convinced most folks will soon realize what we know. We're on the cusp of a farming revolution. We have to be.

Folks are finally realizing what we're doing today simply can't last. We're moving too fast and with too little care. Old Ma Nature doesn't like it.

Stick with the good, organic food she makes. You'll be healthier and happier.

She never lies.

Choose This "Miracle Spice" for a Longer Life

Here's something few folks know. It's something that could save your life.

Cancer is not bad luck.

Sure, a diagnosis is bad. It stands to shake us to our core. Father Time uses the disease as one of his most powerful tools.

But there's new research that proves cancer has nothing to do with luck. Getting cancer is not like getting a bad hand in blackjack.

No, the disease is the result of a lifetime of choices.

Choose wisely... and the deadly disease will pass you by. Choose wrong... and Father Time will come knocking sooner than you want.

What's crazy is that, until quite recently, researchers had no idea what choices led us to cancer. Oh sure, cigarettes were an obvious bad choice and so was tearing out asbestos for a living. But now we're learning there are many more day-to-day choices that affect our odds of getting cancer.

Many of them focus on our diet.

The Doc's Surprise

In fact, there's new research that hints at how the array of bacteria in our gut dictates our overall health.

Get this... A team of doctors recently discovered that a popular chemotherapy drug may work for a previously unknown reason.

It turns out that as the cocktail of chemicals is poured into the body, it does great damage to the layer of mucus that lines our intestine. As the barrier breaks down, gut bacteria are let into the bloodstream.

From there they travel into our lymph nodes... and activate a response from our immune system.

To prove the theory, doctors gave mice an antibiotic to kill that strain of bacteria. That way, there was no chance it could leak out of their guts and into their bloodstreams.

Those mice saw virtually no positive effect from the chemotherapy treatment.

In other words, it wasn't the chemicals saving lives... it was the bacteria.

It's crazy. It's why so many folks these days are obsessed with the flora in the digestive system. Having the right bacteria in the right amounts could mean the difference between life and death.

And, of course, getting things right down there hinges almost entirely on making the right choices.

The Best Decision You Can Make

Getting a bit of **ginger** (*Zingiber officinale* – or what I like to call "Element Z") into our bodies may just be the best decision we can make each day.

I've spent a lot of hours researching the topic. I've looked at journals. I've talked with doctors. But nothing convinced me of the powerful effects of ginger like one piece of data that I just happened to uncover. It turns out there's one country on the planet that consumes more "Element Z" than any other.

In fact, per person, India consumes nearly twice as much ginger as the next highest country. And here's the stunner...

India has some of the lowest cancer rates on the planet.

Take prostate cancer, for instance. Here in the States, it's seemingly everywhere. Out of 100,000 men, 104.3 will be diagnosed with the quiet killer.

But in India... that number is just four.

That's right, in the country that consumes the most ginger, men are 96% less likely to end up with prostate cancer.

And that's not all. Compared with Indians, Americans get...

- Eight to 14 times the rate of melanoma...
- As much as 11 times more colorectal cancer...
- Nine times more endometrial cancer...
- Seventeen times more lung cancer...
- Eight times more bladder cancer...
- Five times more breast cancer...
- As much as 12 times more kidney cancer.

Of course, we can't say for sure it's the ginger.

Indians also eat a lot of turmeric. But thanks to recent research, there's a growing group of folks (yours truly included) who think ginger may be the new miracle spice.

The Miracle Spice

The list of ailments ginger has long been known to prevent, treat or minimize is extensive.

Its anti-inflammatory properties reduce pain and inflammation related to arthritis and rheumatism. It's been shown to boost circulation. Ginger helps rid the body of toxins. It even helps treat fevers and respiratory problems.

Again, it's why we try to consume a bit of it each day. But it's the root's effects on our digestive systems that deserve far more attention than mainstream health experts are giving them.

As the folks at the University of Texas showed, it helps "smooth" our guts and make them work better and more efficiently.

That's a critical idea, given a largely unknown fact – that one-third of cancer develops as a result of our diet. Therefore, what we put into our mouth and what our body does with it plays a huge role in our long-term health.

Again, cancer isn't a bad case of luck. It has everything to do with what we put into – or what gets into – our bodies.

Like an Exterminator for Your Gut

Take a nasty little bacterium called *Helicobacter pylori*. About two-thirds of all humans have the bug living in their bodies.

For a lot of folks, the bacteria don't do much harm. They can live in our bodies for years without being noticed.

But start eating the wrong foods or treating your body poorly and *H. pylori* bacteria can flourish in your stomach. When they do, they will attack your stomach lining, which can lead to ulcers and infection.

What's astonishing is *H. pylori* was the first bacterium on the planet to be listed as a Group 1 carcinogen – meaning that it definitely causes cancer.

Again… it's in most of us right now. But the folks at the University of Illinois recently proved that ginger is the bacteria's natural enemy. In each case studied, ginger was shown to inhibit the growth of the deadly bacteria.

The result was clear.

"These data provide a direct mechanism of action for ginger," the researchers concluded, "and further support its role as a chemopreventative agent."

In other words, thanks to its work in our gut, ginger can prevent cancer.

But it gets better. You see, there are essentially two types of cancer cells. Most cells are the fast-growing type. They are what most modern medicine attacks.

To date, popular cancer drugs like Taxol have not been successful treating the second type of cancer cells… the stem cells.

These pivotal cells represent just 0.2% of all cancer cells, and yet they are some of the toughest to eradicate.

They can self-renew… they're resistant to chemotherapeutic drugs… they're self-sufficient… and they aren't influenced by what's happening to the cells around them.

In a word, they're deadly.

But a new study published by the Public Library of Science revealed that a compound in ginger known as 6-shogaol effectively targets and kills cancerous stem cells.

In fact, this natural ingredient is believed to be as much as 10,000 times more effective than traditional chemotherapy techniques.

Given that fact alone, wouldn't you want to add a bit of ginger to your diet every day?

I could go on and on with the research.

Ginger helps prevent diabetes. It's been shown to lower cholesterol. It helps with Alzheimer's and Parkinson's disease. It's been used to cure migraines. It's even been shown to boost cognitive function and attention span.

Again, superfoods like ginger prove that cancer isn't bad luck. It's the result of all the tiny choices we make during the day – what we put into our body and what we leave out.

Adding a bit of ginger to your daily diet could be one of the best choices you make.

It doesn't take much. Most experts recommend about 4 grams of ground ginger daily. That's about two teaspoons.

You can drink it in a tea, add it to your favorite recipe or, as I recommend, drink it in a delicious and oh-so-healthy glass of my perfect drink (keep reading).

Try it for a month and you'll feel the results. It's a healthy choice.

Nature's Golden Wonder Drug

I t's one of the hottest health trends on the planet. The world is finally figuring out what we've known for a long time... that honey is nature's wonder drug.

But what's crazy is this isn't a new cure.

In fact, the Bible is chock-full of references to honey. It's mentioned at least 61 times.

But it's what God said in Deuteronomy 6 that has us referring to honey as Canaan's Cure. He told Jacob to seek the land of milk and honey.

It was meant as a sign of abundance and good health. And it worked. Jacob lived to be 147 years old.

We now know the health effects of honey are off the charts:

- It contains vitamins B1, B2, B6, C, D and E, plus calcium, iron, potassium and magnesium.

- It fights the "bad" bacteria in your gut and promotes "good" bacteria.

- Raw honey helps boost your immune system by removing free radicals from your body.

- It has antibacterial properties (rub some on your next cut).
- Phytonutrients found in honey have been shown to help prevent certain types of cancer.
- Raw, local honey is thought to fight allergies.

Not to mention it has been shown to fight inflammation, tackle respiratory ailments, tame diabetes and fight chronic insomnia.

All this and it's also one of the most delicious organic substances on the planet. It's sweet with a hint of spice... like what a fine wine should taste like.

Just a spoonful will light up your senses in a way you've likely never experienced.

But the latest craze isn't for the sort of honey we're all used to. No, this time health experts are going gaga over a little-known form of honey that comes almost solely from a tiny sliver of the planet.

This island's honey can't be found anywhere else. And folks are draining their wallets to get their hands on the stuff.

Where a pound of standard clover honey from the States might cost you $12, the same amount of New Zealand's manuka honey might cost you $40 or more.

To understand why there's such a huge difference in price, you need to understand a bit about how bees make honey.

It's fascinating.

Whence It Came

By now, it should be clear that not all honey is the same. In fact, the final product has very little to do with the bees and a whole lot to do with the trees and plants that surround the hive.

Put some bees in a field of clover and you'll get light, sweet honey.

Put them near a field of buckwheat and you'll get dark, bitter honey.

And put them in a forest surrounded by the fragrant, pink flowers of manuka trees that grow only in New Zealand and you'll get what so many folks are paying big bucks for.

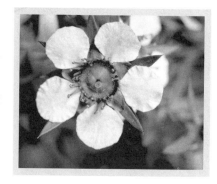

It all has to do with the chemical composition of the nectar produced by various plants. When it comes to manuka, the key ingredient is an enzyme called methylglyoxal (MGO). Manuka honey has more of it than any other form of honey... much more.

The best way to think of MGO is as one of the planet's strongest natural antibiotics.

It's so strong, in fact, that some doctors are now turning to it instead of modern medicine. After all, scientists have yet to find a bacterium that has the ability to grow resistance to it.

While folks are dying from drug-resistant infections and modern medicine's inability to fight back, manuka honey has been quietly hiding in the remote mountains of New Zealand.

But the secret is out, and things are changing fast.

Now hospital bandages are coming soaked in the stuff. Doctors are rubbing it onto their patients' wounds. And superbug infections are on the decline. For folks with serious skin infections, manuka honey is a savior.

Take the story of Alan Partridge, for example.

He was a powerful Olympian and one of England's top marathoners. But back in January of 1999, he came down with flu-like symptoms. At first, he didn't think much of it. But the pain kept getting worse and worse, until...

Twelve hours after his first tinge of pain, he was on life support.

The pain got so bad, his doctors had no choice but to put him in a medically induced coma.

And Alan stayed that way until his doctors were able to amputate his lower legs and most of his fingers.

Even after doctors put their saws away, Alan wasn't out of the woods. Nine months later, his wounds still refused to heal. He got one skin graft after the next.

That's when Alan found out about some research from New Zealand's University of Waikato... that detailed the immense healing effects of manuka honey.

The doctors involved in the study were stunned.

"The results have proven the existence of a formerly secret synergist," they wrote.

As soon as he heard that renowned doctors realized they had a miracle cure on their hands, Alan went all-in.

He got his hands on manuka honey and gave it a try.

The turnaround was miraculous.

"After nine months with no healing," Alan said, "within nine weeks, they had completely healed. Just like that."

Just like that... manuka honey attacked and killed the superbugs that were threatening to send a young man to his grave.But this incredible story doesn't mean you should go pushing traditional honey aside.

After all, many of the beneficial properties of MGO are lost when our body's digestive system gets done with its job.

After digestion, manuka honey and various other forms of (cheaper) honey are on par with each other.

In other words, the miracles happen before the stuff gets to our gut – like on our skin and in our throats.

That means manuka is a superior skin treatment, is better at fighting the nasty germs that cause strep throat and the common cold, and is a leader when it comes to treating sinus issues.

But be warned... not all manuka sold in the States is worthy of the high price tags.

What to Buy

As happens with things related to a craze, there are lots of folks looking to take advantage of excited buyers who are desperate for some help.

Fortunately, there are some easy things that will tell you whether you're buying the real deal.

First, there should be one or two numbers on every bottle of manuka honey. If you don't see these numbers, don't buy it.

The first number represents the MGO level. It tells us how much of the special enzyme is present in the honey. It's measured in milligrams per kilogram. Look for anything higher than 260.

The next number measures the same thing, just a bit differently. The honey's non-peroxide activity (NPA) is measured as a total percentage of the overall composition. Look for an NPA figure of 10 or higher.

If the numbers are lower, there may be manuka present in the honey, but it's not enough to show any real medicinal benefit. Don't buy it.

The bottom line is if you have a skin condition or feel like you may be getting sick, a bit of manuka honey may fix what ails you.

But when it comes to the many benefits of ingesting a spoonful of honey, traditional honey is just as good.

The Ancient Elixir With Amazing Powers

Cleopatra must have been quite a woman. By all accounts, she lived a life of luxury. Ancient works tell of her lying around, nearly naked, covered in jewels.

Many of those jewels, the books tell us, were pearls. The Egyptian ruler was flat-out obsessed with the dainty little things.

She had lots of them... but there are just two worth spilling ink about today. Those pearls lead us to some of the most powerful medicine on Earth.

You see, Cleopatra owned the two largest pearls the world had ever seen. Early experts put their worth at some 60 million sestertii (ancient Roman coins)... or about $28.5 million in today's dollars.

But money wasn't much of a concern for the lusty lady... and she was eager to prove it to her powerful Roman lover. Working to secure the eye of Mark Antony and highlight the wealth of her land, Cleopatra made a bet.

She bet she could host the most expensive dinner in history.

Up for a good show, Antony took the bet and watched as she crushed one of those magnificent, multimillion-dollar pearls, tossed it into a glass of liquid and consumed it all in one big gulp.

What's odd is that I first heard this tale not from a history book or some dark hallway in a museum... but from a doctor – a doc who was reciting the rich history of a not-so-understood elixir.

Thanks to Cleopatra's bold move, I call the powerful liquid Pearl's Milk... but most folks know it simply as **apple cider vinegar** (ACV).

History's Best-Kept Secret

The Egyptian ruler certainly wasn't the first person to note the power of the acidic juice. In fact, the father of all medicine, Hippocrates, supposedly wrote one of the world's first-ever prescriptions around 400 B.C... telling his sick patient to drink a bit of ACV.

If the history books have it right, the ancient doc used ACV to treat some 17 ailments, ranging from ulcers and digestion to skin problems.

From there, the power of the unique chemical concoction remained well-known for centuries. Columbus, in fact, made sure that each of his ships had several barrels of ACV on it.

It was used to prevent scurvy and keep his sailors in the best shape possible... despite some of the worst conditions possible.

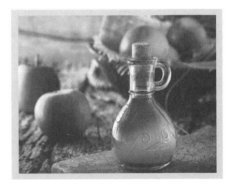

Japanese samurais, too, praised the liquid for its powers... and Civil War doctors ordered the stuff to help treat the wounded.

But it's the modern-day uses and case studies that have our attention.

Despite modern medicine's tendency to focus on new, higher-priced drugs, the power of ACV remains well-known in a few (growing) underground circles.

Take a fellow named Don Wilders, for instance. When he had a heart attack at age 46, he thought his life was over.

The clock was ticking. The next one could kill him. And it could come any day.

That was way back in the 1950s. And Don ended up living quite a long life. He recently passed away at the ripe old age of 96.

Until the day he died, he swore his late-life health came thanks to one thing... his daily ritual of drinking just two tablespoons of ACV.

We have every reason to believe him.

Nature's Fix-It-All

Recent studies have quietly shown that a small daily dose of ACV can lower blood pressure... slash cholesterol... and reduce triglycerides – the fats from our liver that are a leading culprit in deadly heart disease.

There aren't many studies available on ACV (Big Pharma's not a fan of the stuff, after all), but I was able to get my hands on a few.

One comes to us from the Central Research Group in Aichi, Japan.

It found that ACV was able to reduce systolic blood pressure by an amazing 20 mmHG over the course of just six weeks.

To further test the merits of what many consider the world's oldest medicine, the same group also fed a group of rats a diet loaded with cholesterol.

From there, one half of the group was given a daily allotment of ACV.

The other received none.

And just as we'd expect... the group given the vinegar came out far healthier – with greatly reduced cholesterol and triacylglycerol levels.

The researchers concluded that ACV stops what's called lipogenesis – the process in which our body turns sugar into fat.

That's huge.

Imagine drinking a couple of tablespoons of ACV each day... and telling your body to stop making fat.

Your Sugar Fix

This ancient elixir is also believed to be beneficial for folks dealing with diabetes.

In fact, doctors at Arizona State University recently put ACV to the test in a study detailed in the official journal of the American Diabetes Association.

The scientists wanted to determine whether drinking just two tablespoons a day would lead to improved glucose levels.

It did.

Fasting glucose was lowered by 4%, with folks at higher initial glucose levels seeing an average drop of 6%.

Here's what the research concluded:

> *These data suggest that vinegar ingestion at bedtime may favorably impact waking glucose concentrations in type 2 diabetes. The antiglycemic effect of acetic acid, the active ingredient in vinegar, has been attributed to reduced starch digestion and/or delayed gastric emptying.*

But this is where skeptical folks should pay attention.

The study also pointed out that the standard treatment from Big Pharma lowered glucose levels by 10% to 15%... but those participants had significantly higher starting levels.

It proves that, while ACV may not be quite as potent as long-term drug therapy, it's certainly competitive.... and doesn't have nearly the same level of side effects.

To see why that's important, we turn not to the esteemed Harvard School of Medicine... but to the Harvard Center for Ethics.

In a scathing report, the Ivy League group starts with a bold fact.

"Few people know that new prescription drugs have a 1 in 5 chance of causing serious reactions after they have been approved," writes the school's institutional corruption expert Dr. Donald Light. "That is why expert physicians recommend not taking new drugs for at least five years unless patients have first tried better-established options and have the need to do so."

He goes on... opening our eyes with some scary facts:

- A recent review of American hospital charts shows that even *properly prescribed* drugs lead to big trouble – causing 1.9 million hospitalizations each year.

- Some 840,000 people are given drugs that cause serious adverse reactions each year.

- From those figures, 128,000 Americans die annually from drugs prescribed to them.

- Combined, these factors make legally prescribed drugs the fourth leading cause of death.

Those are numbers Big Pharma definitely does not want you to see.

We won't be naïve and forget that prescription drugs save many, many more lives each year. That would be ignorant and would be dangerously flawed logic.

But it certainly makes sense to seek natural and healthy alternatives that will get the job done... and aren't loaded with surprise side effects.

That's the proven value of ACV.

For many folks, taking just a bit of ACV each day could mean the difference between adding another prescription to their daily routine and staying pill-free for many more years.

With just a bit of ACV by itself or as part of the Perfect Drink (next chapter) each morning, your body could be running as smoothly and pain-free as it did when you were just 18 years old... before decades of stress and strain took their toll.

Get the Good Stuff

Perhaps the best thing about ACV and the ultimate reason Big Pharma wants nothing to do with it is it's cheap... dirt cheap.

And there's no money in cheap medicine.

Many folks make ACV at home. But even the most expensive of store-bought varieties is still dirt cheap... running just a few bucks for a supply that will last months.

But not all ACV is created equally.

The good stuff – the raw and unpasteurized vinegar – is filled with healthy bacteria and nutrients that help to greatly boost its health effects.

To get your hands on this product, look for unfiltered and unpasteurized ACV. Most often, it will be organic.

Non-organic, filtered ACV (which will likely be clear but not colorless) is fine. It still offers plenty of health-boosting potential. It's just not as beneficial as the natural product.

That's the key with this potent medicine... It's natural.

Just two tablespoons of ACV a day have been proven to have magical effects on your body – that are the near equivalent of Big Pharma's answer to what ails us.

When it comes to ACV, the studies are clear. And the stories are true.

Cleopatra used it to win a bet.

Now you should use apple cider vinegar to improve your health.

Feel Better and More Energized With the Perfect Drink

T he old-timers knew what they were doing. They created what could be considered the ultimate health drink... long before such things were a fad.

This fascinating drink cuts inflammation, quenches thirst, restores muscle and offers an energy boost that rivals a cup of coffee's. These days, though, few folks have ever heard of it.

Instead, modern store shelves are filled with dangerous energy drinks pumped with chemicals, additives and artificial colors. While they represent great marketing efforts, these drinks are hardly something healthy to put into our bodies.

For that, we turn to a centuries-old drink – a drink with a short, all-natural list of ingredients that's bound to leave you feeling better and more energized. We call it **haymaker punch**, but it goes by several other names, like switchel and switzel.

Drink This... Feel Better

As far as we can tell, variations of the drink have been around nearly as long as humans have known of the benefits of fermenting.

But the version below came to North America through the West Indies sometime in the 1600s. Once American hardworking farmers discovered the rejuvenating effects of the beverage, it became an instant hit.

The ingredient list for haymaker punch is simple. Everything needed is already in our cupboards.

- Ginger
- Honey or molasses
- Apple cider vinegar

To the uninitiated, it sounds like a bad joke. But mix the ingredients in the right proportions (see recipe on Page 35), and the sweet and tangy flavor will instantly change your mind.

Even so, Manward rewards function over form. While haymaker punch is pleasant on the palate, it's what it does for our bodies that gets the nod from us.

The Right Stuff

The addition of ginger is what sets the drink apart from a millennia-old drink known as posca (the drink many say gave the Roman army its enemy-crushing energy).

The root was quite expensive and uncommon in 17th-century Europe, but as settlers moved through the Caribbean, where ginger is easily grown, prices dropped and its popularity soared.

It was quickly added to posca's simple ingredient list... and haymaker punch was born.

Ginger, our miracle spice, has immense value as an ingredient in our tonic.

It fights inflammation. It offers painkilling properties that rival over-the-counter medicines. It boosts immunity. And, finally, anybody who's ever been seasick knows just a bit of ginger can quickly calm an upset stomach.

And that's just one ingredient.

Apple cider vinegar also plays a vital role in haymaker punch.

It is nature's great equalizer.

Just a tablespoon or two of apple cider vinegar each day helps to balance the acidity of your stomach – reducing acid reflux and other painful issues. It helps maintain healthy cholesterol levels. It balances your blood sugar, boosts energy levels... and its high levels of potassium cut leg cramps.

And let's not forget our favorite ingredient... honey.

Packed with vitamins B1, B2, B6, C, D and E, plus calcium, iron, potassium and magnesium, this miraculous substance fights the "bad" bacteria in your gut and promotes "good" bacteria.

These three ingredients combine to offer powerful antioxidants that also help fight dementia and Alzheimer's. With health-boosting properties like these, it's no surprise to see haymaker punch starting to gain some popularity again. I saw it recently at a local market.

But you don't need to buy this ultra-healthy tonic – especially an expensive version at a farmers market. You can make it at home in just a few minutes... for just a few pennies.

Try a glass each day, and watch as your body starts to reward you for feeding it a good, healthy drink.

It's time to bring back a classic.

Recipe for the Perfect Drink

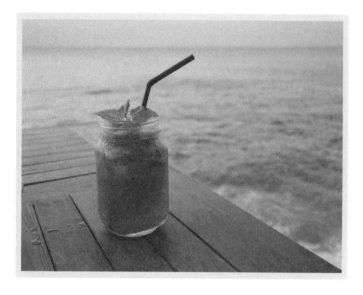

Haymaker's Punch

2 quarts water

1/2 cup apple cider vinegar

3/4 cup honey

1/2 tablespoon ground ginger

Simply combine the ingredients, stir them well and pour a tall glass over ice. For a variation, substitute the water with some seltzer.

Get What Your Body Needs With the Perfect Food

This is the first time we've fully detailed what we believe to be the perfect food.

Men love this topic because, for once, we're not being told to eat a tasteless, far-from-filling salad.

Nope, the perfect food... the *best* healthy food to eat... is the lowly **potato**.

Get this...

Andrew Taylor recently made waves in the nutrition world when he vowed to eat only potatoes for a year.

The carb-counting crowd thought the 36-year-old Australian was nuts.

But it turns out he knew what he was doing.

"I feel amazing. Everything is going real well," Taylor said four months into his diet. "I've got a lot of energy. I'm sleeping better. I've lost a lot of weight."

Those are big words for a man fighting a self-described food addiction.

And don't think Taylor was sacrificing taste to find health and lose dozens of pounds. He topped many of his helpings – which included mashed potatoes and sweet potatoes – with barbecue sauce, herbs and other sensible flavorings.

He even drank a few beers while on the diet.

Power-Packin' Potatoes

There's no doubt potatoes have gotten a bad rap over the last decade. It's mainly their carbohydrate content that's to blame.

But researchers are eager to tell us there's much more to a spud than its carb count.

For example, we've all heard that bananas are a go-to source of potassium – an important vitamin that's typically quite low in the average American's diet. But you'd have to eat four bananas to get the same amount of potassium you'd find in just one potato.

It's the same thing with fiber...

Move over, prunes. A typical potato contains 7 grams of fiber. That's more than a couple slices of bread.

But it doesn't stop there. Potatoes contain at least some of every vital nutrient... things like iron, copper, manganese, vitamin C and several critical forms of vitamin B.

In other words, if our body needs it, it's in a potato – good news for Taylor.

And, for dieters, potatoes have another trick up their sleeve. They tend to leave us fuller, faster.

The so-called "satiety value" of a potato is off the charts. It's higher than any other food that's been tested.

So if you don't feel full after eating a salad, scrape the lettuce off your plate and replace it with a potato. And here's another little-known fact... a bit of Manward myth-busting, if you will...

Lots of folks believe sweet potatoes are healthier than a typical white potato. With one little exception, <u>it's not true</u>.

The main difference is that sweet potatoes are a bit lower on the glycemic index. That means they release their carbs into our bloodstream at a slower pace, resulting in a lower spike in blood sugar than we'd get from a typical potato.

Other than that, there isn't a whole lot of difference between the varieties. So when folks ask us what's the best healthy food to eat... we say it's the humble white potato.

What's Cooking?

Of course, how we cook our potatoes matters. As with anything, a bit of common sense must prevail.

Frying potatoes in a bath of high-fat oil is a lousy idea. Instead, bake or roast them with the skins on. And don't smother them in butter or other not-so-healthy toppings. Toss on a bit of garlic or just a dash of salt to spice them up.

And perhaps one of the very best aspects of potatoes is they make an excellent survival food. It's why we always have a bucket of potatoes in the pantry... with many more in the ground.

If the need should come, we'd survive just fine on the odd-looking tubers. We might, like Taylor has, even find ourselves in better shape.

We'd rather not eat the perfect food for every meal of every day, but it's nice to know we could.

This $2.48 Snack Could Extend Your Life

We love it when health experts get caught up in semantics. It shows just how simple – er, dumb – humans can be.

You see, when it comes to **peanuts**, the debate isn't whether they are good for us or not.

They are.

The debate is about whether they can be compared to more high-brow tree nuts like almonds, cashews and walnuts. Food snobs are quick to point out that peanuts aren't actually nuts. They're legumes – just like soybeans and peas.

We say phooey... it's nonsense.

The fact is that peanuts – whether they have the same high-dollar price tag as a fancy tin of cashews or not – are one of the healthiest foods on the planet.

Caviar? No. Healthy? You Bet!

It's especially true when it comes to heart health.

Peanuts offer an ideal all-around mix of nutrition and appetite-suppressing fiber.

But any discussion of the "legume" must start with fat.

Many folks will tell you that peanuts are chock-full of fat. The less informed will tell you to avoid them because of it.

They're wrong.

Yes, they're high in fat (about 50% of the overall content)... but it's the good kind of fat.

In fact, peanuts have roughly the same fat profile as oh-so-popular olive oil. They contain roughly 80% unsaturated fat and just 20% saturated fat (and most of that is the heart-friendly monounsaturated fat).

In other words, study after study shows the sorts of fats contained in a handful of peanuts go a long way in reducing cholesterol levels and overall risk of heart disease.

But peanuts aren't good only for our hearts. They're good for our brains, too.

Get this. Folks with low daily folic acid intake have higher associations with a number of nasty ailments. They're more likely to suffer from depression... have heart issues... and develop certain types of cancer.

Studies have shown that we can fight back by simply boosting folic acid intake to about 400 micrograms per day. That's good news for fans of the "lowly" peanut. It's one of the highest sources of folic acid on the planet.

And, as a bonus, folic acid is believed to be an essential element in preventing cognitive decline.

In other words, you're literally smarter for eating peanuts.

Dr. Copper

Finally, there's one oft-overlooked mineral that's packed into every peanut. It doesn't get nearly enough attention from the health press.

Copper is essential to our good health.

It helps maintain our energy production and the activity in our brain. Our neurons need a healthy dose of copper to create and protect the axons that make our brains work efficiently.

If we don't get enough of the stuff, big trouble ensues.

Recent research shows that a lack of copper appears to play a leading role in nasty brain conditions, including Alzheimer's and Parkinson's disease.

Beyond the brain, studies have shown that even mild levels of copper deficiency can lead to heart disease and high cholesterol levels.

The simple way to prevent a deficiency – and ensure you get enough heart-healthy fats and folic acid – is to simply eat a handful or two of peanuts each day.

A quarter of a cup is all it takes to take full advantage of this "lowly" legume.

And rest assured... it pairs quite well with our Perfect Drink (see Page 35).

Save Room for the Perfect Dessert

We hope you've been saving room. We've got the recipe for the perfect after-dinner treat.

It contains three main ingredients: **yogurt**, **chia seeds** and **blueberries**.

All three have merits that must be shared.

We'll start with something so important to some ancient cultures that it was once used as a man's measure of wealth: chia seeds.

Derived from a Central American plant in the mint family, chia seeds have some amazing benefits, especially if you're looking for a natural, long-lasting boost of energy.

Some say the tiny seeds are powerful enough to feed an army.

Indeed, Aztec warriors reportedly ate the seeds before going to battle – touting the fact that just one spoonful could sustain them for 24 hours.

Today, runners are the main proponents of chia seeds.

The tiny bites deliver a massive amount of nutrients with very few calories. They're packed with protein (about 14% of their total weight). They contain more omega-3s than the equivalent weight of salmon.

And a single ounce offers nearly 20% of your body's daily calcium requirement.

A spoonful of chia seeds each day is one of the best things you can do for your body.

Fill 'Er Up

Our next ingredient is yogurt – an ultra-healthy food that most folks are familiar with.

But what you may not know is yogurt is quite a good source of protein. That's good news for folks trying to build or maintain their strength... but it's also a critical factor for folks looking to lose weight.

Protein, scientists now know, is the key trigger to releasing the hormones that tell us our stomach is full.

It's what tells our body when enough is enough.

By ensuring ample protein intake, yogurt naturally keeps us eating less. One study, in fact, showed that yogurt eaters routinely consumed 100 fewer calories per meal.

That's big.

You Should Know This

Our third ingredient gets high marks from the medical crowd. Some even say it's the perfect fruit.

Blueberries have been shown to improve memory... lower blood pressure... reduce depression... cut inflammation... and even lower blood sugar levels.

But it's the tiny fruit's role in cancer treatment that gets our attention.

This is huge.

In a report released almost exactly a year ago (and yet we bet you still haven't heard about it), doctors proved that adding simple blueberry extract to traditional radiation therapy can significantly improve cancer survival rates.

Check out these numbers.

When docs treated cancer cells with radiation alone... they killed 20% of the cells.

And when they treated the same type of cells using only blueberry extract... they killed 25% of cells.

The natural cure was better than the "scientific" cure.

But keep reading...

When the study combined the two treatments, the number of deadly cancer cells plunged by 70%.

So, um, how about some blueberries?

The Recipe for the Perfect Dessert

When we combine these three main ingredients with just a handful of others, we get a delicious dessert or midday snack.

And unlike most processed snack foods today, this one can help extend your life... not shorten it.

It's called **Chia Seed Pudding**.

Here's everything you'll need:

- 1 cup of milk
- 1 cup of yogurt
- 2 tablespoons of maple syrup (or raw honey)

- 1 teaspoon of vanilla extract
- 1/4 cup of chia seeds
- 1 pint of blueberries
- Pinch of salt

To get things started, combine the milk, chia seeds, yogurt, maple syrup, vanilla and salt in a bowl. Whisk them until they're blended. Refrigerate the mixture for eight hours, stirring occasionally to keep the seeds from settling.

The now-thickened pudding is ready to go.

To serve, simply add the blueberries and perhaps a light drizzle of honey, a handful of almonds or a scoop of granola to the top of the dish.

It's a healthy – and delicious – dessert.

Its ingredients prove that good health isn't for folks with good luck.

Good health is for folks who make good decisions.

Recipe for the Perfect Dessert

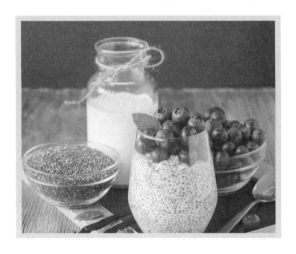

Chia Seed Pudding

1 cup milk

1 cup yogurt

2 tablespoons maple syrup (or raw honey)

1 teaspoon vanilla extract

1/4 cup chia seeds

1 pint blueberries

Pinch of salt

Combine the milk, chia seeds, yogurt, maple syrup, vanilla and salt in a bowl. Whisk them until they're blended. Refrigerate the mixture for eight hours, stirring occasionally to keep the seeds from settling.

To serve, simply add the blueberries and perhaps a light drizzle of honey, a handful of almonds or a scoop of granola to the top of the dish.

A Sweet Treat for Your Health

I t's true that the best things often come in the smallest of packages. We were reminded of the idea last winter when a small package showed up at our front door.

Looking at the label, we found no name but could see that the box was sent to us from Mexico.

Interesting.

We opened it and were surprised by the contents.

Dates. Several pounds of them.

With some sleuthing, we determined the package was sent to us by some friends visiting America's southern neighbor.

They came across a date farm and, after touring it, knew they had to share their discovery with us.

We're sure glad they did.

Nature's Medicine

Despite being virtually ignored by the mainstream press and even many health experts, **dates** are a wonderful food.

Since they were first eaten by humans thousands of years ago, dates have been thought to have immense health effects.

In some cultures, the fruits have a nearly mystical following.

But modern science eliminates any doubt as to their power. Dates are incredibly healthy.

As one of nature's rare foods that contain no cholesterol, dates are a smart way to keep a check on one of the leading forms of heart disease.

But aside from merely containing no cholesterol, dates have another artery-clearing ingredient: potassium, which actually helps our bodies eliminate cholesterol.

The fruit is also quite good for our digestive system.

Many experts say to soak a few dates in water and eat them. The high fiber content helps to ensure everything works as it's supposed to.

And finally, dates are high in iron – an essential mineral.

If you've been feeling tired, sluggish or just plain worn out, it may be because of an iron deficiency.

If your body doesn't have enough iron, it can't make enough oxygen-carrying red blood cells. A few dates each day may help put some spring in your step.

Eat This... Live Longer

Of course, there are lots of ways to eat dates – everything from eating them plain (they're delicious) to wrapping them in bacon.

But my favorite way to eat them turns this nutritious snack into a delicious and incredibly healthy dessert.

Don't let the name of this recipe fool you... there's nothing "fudgy" about these **Fudge Balls**.

They're a healthy and delicious snack.

The recipe, of course, starts with dates. You'll need about seven to 10 of them pitted.

From there, the healthiness continues with half a cup of **cashews** or **walnuts** – both are considered highly heart-healthy foods.

Before mixing with the other ingredients, soak them in water overnight to soften them up.

After that, you'll need two tablespoons of raw **cacao**.

If you're not familiar with this ingredient, you should be. It's considered an "Amazonian Superfood."

It boasts 40 times more antioxidants than blueberries (which is incredible), and it's packed full of iron (the highest levels of any plant) and magnesium.

Plus, it's thought to be one of nature's best antidepressants.

Next, you'll need half a teaspoon each of **cinnamon** (great for the heart) and **vanilla extract** (another great source of antioxidants).

Finally, you'll need a pinch of salt – we recommend Himalayan or sea salt – and seven tablespoons of date water.

The latter is just what it sounds like. It's made by simply soaking your dates in water for 30 minutes or so.

Once the dates and nuts are soaked properly, put all the ingredients in a food processor and blend them until they're the consistency of thick dough.

From there, roll them into something that resembles the size of a golf ball... and toss 'em in the freezer.

Once frozen, they make a delicious and incredibly healthy dessert.

After one bite, you'll be convinced that good things absolutely do come in small packages.

Recipe for the Perfect Treat

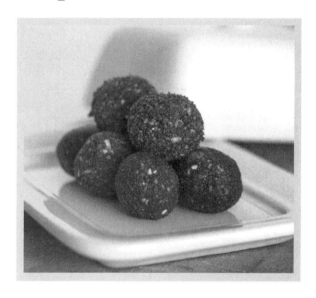

Fudge Balls

7 to **10** pitted dates (soak for 30 minutes)

1/2 cup cashews (soak overnight)

2 tablespoons raw cacao

1/2 teaspoon cinnamon

1/2 teaspoon vanilla extract

Pinch of salt

Combine ingredients in a food processor and blend until they're the consistency of thick dough. Roll into balls and freeze.

The Lowly Weed That Fights Cancer

Here's a sad fact. The average American can recognize the logos of thousands of commercial brands. And yet they can identify fewer than five plants growing in their area.

In other words, little Johnny is more likely to recognize the logo on his Apple phone... than the leaves of a real apple tree.

Scary.

But the miraculous plant we're about to tell you about – a plant that's believed to have the power to renew our liver, help control diabetes and even slow the growth of cancer – is one we all recognize.

First brought here by the Pilgrims and now considered a lowly weed that's eradicated on sight by many American homeowners, "Pilgrim's Herb" was once a welcome visitor in yards around the world. Until the 1800s, in fact, folks actually pulled the grass from their yards to make room for it.

Before the age of Big Pharma, these folks knew what was good for them.

You may never have heard of a plant dubbed the Pilgrim's Herb.

But perhaps you've heard the French name "dent de lion." It translates to "lion's tooth."

Say it fast enough, and you'll know we're talking about the lowly **dandelion**... that yellow-petaled weed American gardeners spend big time and big money trying to eradicate from their yards.

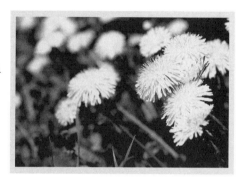

It's a mistake.

The dandelion shouldn't be covered with herbicide and left to wither and die. Oh no.

If folks knew its true power, they'd grow fields of the stuff.

Researchers' Delight

It seems the more scientists study the health effects of the lowly dandelion, the more they realize just how powerful it is.

Take its ability to fight cancer, for instance. A recent study out of Canada showed that the plant's root extract killed melanoma cells without hurting nearby noncancerous cells.

Another study from folks at the University of Windsor found similar effects on leukemia.

Pamela Ovadje was the lead doctor for that research.

"We had information from an oncologist, a collaborator here in Windsor, who had patients that showed improvement after taking dandelion-root tea," she said.

"And so, with a phone call, we decided to start studying what was in this tea that made patients respond to it, so we started digging up dandelions."

She dubbed the early results "eye-opening" and immediately went all-in on more in-depth studies.

She's not the only one... and it's not just cancer docs who are getting surprised by the power of dandelions.

Another study recently showed that dandelions have a similar effect on the body as the popular prescription weight loss drug orlistat. Both work to slow or stop the release of pancreatic lipase, an enzyme our bodies use to break down fat.

And research last year suggests that the unique polysaccharides (a chief source of energy) in dandelions help to increase the function of the liver and rid it of harmful toxins.

We could go on about the potential effects of dandelions.

We've heard of folks claiming they're good for digestion... urinary function... skin problems... blood pressure... circulation... and even poor vision.

But we imagine most readers don't need more benefits... they want to know how to take advantage of them.

It's easy.

Drink Up

Most folks find it a bit surprising – after all, our culture seems to be at war with the weed – but it's safe to eat a whole dandelion right out of the ground.

Of course, that's assuming the plant has been washed and has never been treated by fertilizer or an herbicide.

Dandelions make a great addition to a salad or even a garnish on meat. And its sweet taste is a natural appetite suppressant.

To find plants that are safe to eat, we recommend heading to a good local grocer that specializes in health food.

Another popular option is to make dandelion tea.

Simply steep the roots and/or flower of the plant in boiling water for 30 minutes or so. Some folks strain the plant from the water, but we say let it stay. That way nothing goes to waste.

Dandelion coffee is a bit more complex... but it's still quite easy.

To make a delicious coffee substitute (it doesn't contain caffeine but does offer a more natural boost of energy), you'll need to chop up the dandelion root and roast it in an oven set at 300 degrees for about two hours.

After that, make it the same way you would a normal cup of coffee.

But before we put our pen down, we must answer what is perhaps the top question asked by everybody we share this information with.

"Why didn't I know this?"

Folks want to know why the benefits of dandelions aren't well-known.

We say we already answered that question.

Dandelions are everywhere. Unlike the "traditional" medicine we stuff into our bodies, we don't need to pay for the plant. It grows right out our back door.

Therefore, there's no money in dandelions.

If Big Pharma finds out we're growing an alternative to its dope right in our backyard – entirely by accident – it's going to be none too happy. Quarterly profits are going to sink.

It'd rather we eradicate them with our Saturday morning fertilizer applications.

That way it gets paid... and its branding stays fresh in our minds.

Forget that stuff. Get some lion's tooth in your diet.

If you don't feel like harvesting your own, hop on over to Amazon where you can buy all you need for as little as $4.72.

The Drink That Fuels the World

W e're told beer is the fuel that changed the world.

If it weren't for their low stores of beer, the story goes, the Pilgrims wouldn't have stopped at Plymouth Rock.

Beer is what made the water safe to drink in many classical European towns.

And there are even rumors that, perhaps, the amber gift of the gods was the motivation for the great pyramids.

We don't doubt all that.

But we do argue that beer's only half the story. After all, where there's a night filled with beer, there's a morning filled with coffee.

It, too, is a bit of a wonder drink. There are immense health benefits to drinking **coffee**.

According to the fine folks at Harvard, coffee can cut the risk of Parkinson's disease nearly in half, can fight against heart disease and diabetes, and has even been shown to reduce depression.

It's why we drink a cup with breakfast and then slowly sip another cup or so from our thermos throughout the day.

The Downside

But this supposed miracle nectar doesn't come without some side effects. Coffee can wreak havoc on your gut... a region of the body doctors are finding is more important to our overall health than we once realized.

A lot of folks drink coffee on an empty stomach. They roll out of bed and head right for the coffee pot.

It's bad news...

Putting nothing but coffee in your stomach triggers your body to produce hydrochloric acid, creating an environment that's ripe for trouble.

The combination of caffeine, catechols and a couple of other complex chemicals kick-starts a chain reaction of trouble.

It causes us to be more prone to ulcers, it weakens the vital mucosal layer and it creates a breeding ground for the bad bacteria that lead to digestive problems.

In fact, some 40 million people in the U.S. suffer from coffee-induced stomach problems. It's coffee's downfall.

Fortunately, there's a simple solution.

It's why our cupboard has a unique kind of coffee from Folgers (look for the green "Simply Smooth" label) that's roasted in a way that reduces key stomach irritants.

The taste is noticeably milder, but after just a few pots, your body will want nothing else.

If Folgers isn't your brand, there's a growing number of stomach-friendly roasts on the market.

The Myths

To be sure, coffee has had its enemies over the years. Some of them led us to myths that stubbornly persist today.

Certainly all of us have heard the idea that coffee stunts growth.

It's bunk.

Most of today's kids won't touch the stuff, but if they did drink coffee, it would have no effect on their height. In fact, we can chalk this myth up to yet another aggressive advertising campaign.

Begin Early—

Children "brought up" on

POSTUM

are free from the evil effects of caffeine—the habit-forming drug—in coffee and tea.

Postum is made of clean, hard wheat, skillfully roasted, including the bran-coat which contains the Phosphate of Potash (grown in the grain) for building healthy brain and nerve tissue.

Begin early to insure a healthy nervous system for the little ones.

"There's a Reason"

Iced Postum—served with sugar and lemon is a delicious, cooling Summer food-drink.

Postum Cereal Co., Ltd., Battle Creek, Mich. U. S. A.

The legend supposedly started when cereal tycoon C.W. Post railed against coffee after introducing a coffee alternative called Postum – made out of wheat, bran and molasses.

Post launched a nasty campaign against coffee, using fake science to scare adults and children away from the drink.

He said by crowding milk out of their diet, coffee-drinking kids become malnourished, sluggish and... short.

As usual, time has told the truth. It turns out the only thing wrong with giving coffee to kids is that, well, you'll have a highly caffeinated kid – reason alone to forbid the stuff.

The New Health Benefits of Coffee

Thanks to more recent research, though, you may start to see coffee and its key ingredient caffeine in products that go *on* your body, not in it.

A lot of skin care products are now adding caffeine to their lists of ingredients, as it's been shown to tighten skin, reduce inflammation and, get this, reduce bulging fat.

A recent study showed that 76% of folks who used a caffeine-based fat-burning cream saw the circumference of their thighs shrink by an average of half an inch.

There's no word on what it can do for a beer belly... But caffeine has shown a similar effect on dark, puffy circles under the eyes.

That's science you can use next time you have a few too many beers.

Bottom line: Beer may get all the attention. But coffee is truly the drink that keeps the world moving.

Drink up... and don't feel guilty.

Feed Your Gut and Fight Infection

I t's no secret that America has a problem with antibiotics. They're overprescribed, misused and increasingly ineffective.

Part of the problem is that our society has become sterile. Not only is the truth being whitewashed until the nightly news is entirely inoffensive, but so is everything around us.

We wash our hands in little more than fine-smelling bleach. We wipe our countertops with chemicals that could kill a cow. And, the silent killer, our food is as dead as the paper we read each morning.

This Superfood Brings Out the Health Within Us

Nearly half of the food ingested by modern man is dead. The vitamins have been refined out. The fiber and minerals are all but gone. But it sure does taste good... and leaves us wanting more.

The list of "dead" food is long.

Bread. Pasta. Sugar. Frozen meals. Fried food. Most of the stuff you'd find on a cheap restaurant menu.

It's perfectly possible to live on these foods... especially if you don't mind standing in line for your drugs.

Fortunately (certainly it's not coincidental), we conquered the realm of modern medicine just as we mastered the art of processing our food.

But there is a better way.

Perhaps it's the 20/20 vision of hindsight, but many doctors and scientists are now realizing that the diets of our ancestors were far better at fighting off ailments than we realized.

Really, we don't have to go all that far back in history to see the idea at work.

In the 1950s, for example, Europe was struck by an epidemic of typhoid.

Few things seemed able to slow it down.

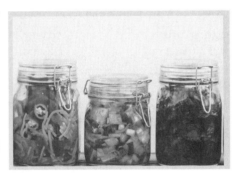

But then astute observers realized that fresh sauerkraut – **a fermented food** that's alive with beneficial bacteria – was quite effective at killing off the bad bacteria that caused typhoid.

Later, scientists realized that a naturally occurring strain of lactic acid found in sourdough bread is surprisingly effective at killing the deadly superbugs that are increasingly resistant to modern antibiotics.

Doctors following the development are astonished the mainstream world of medicine hasn't caught on to the powerful effects of food that's "alive" with beneficial bugs.

Then again, these are likely the same pharmaceutical-backed docs pushing high-priced opioids.

It's a whole lot easier for Big Pharma to make a buck or two selling antibiotics than it is to push a good sauerkraut recipe.

The Health Within Us

The truth is that as much as 70% of our immune system is based in our gut. That means when we kill the good bacteria that live in our gut by eating dead, processed foods, we're taking a dagger directly to the delicate system that keeps us healthy.

Dead food is cheap, easy and convenient, but it destroys our body's ability to fight for itself.

It forces us to rely on modern medicine and pills that are becoming less effective with each meal.

Instead of eating dead food, we must eat food that's rich in the sort of good bacteria that feeds our healthy gut... probiotics.

Recent research by *The American Journal of Clinical Nutrition* used big words to sum it up.

"Probiotic bacteria are shown to promote the endogenous host defense mechanisms... [and] stimulate nonspecific host resistance to microbial pathogens."

In other words... good bacteria beats bad bacteria.

As the Germans taught us, fermented foods – like sauerkraut, pickles, raw cheese, yogurt and kefir – are far better at keeping us healthy than many modern chemicals.

Our culture may be trying to sterilize all that we do and eat... but we must resist it.

We'll be a whole lot healthier.

The Ideal Menu for Better Brain Function

V anity is an evil beast. Drive through any urban or suburban neighborhood, and you're bound to pass a few gyms.

Inside, folks are huffing, puffing and dripping sweat in the name of looking good. Oh sure, they'll tell us they're doing it for their health – and some genuinely are.

But for most of the 20- and 30-somethings wiping their brows, it's a lie that even they don't truly believe.

If health were their first concern, we argue, all of America would be practicing a new form of exercise.

It's called **neurobics**.

As its name implies, it's all about exercising your mind.

It's not hard. You'll never break a sweat or find yourself out of breath.

Doing puzzles, reading thought-provoking books and even watching the TV quieter than you normally would are all ample forms of neurobics.

But what most folks forget is that our brain is an organ that relies on some very precise chemistry. And if the mix of chemicals isn't just right, it will never work at its peak efficiency.

Eat This, Think Better

There are all sorts of scientific evidence that proves it: *What we eat affects the way we think.*

Just as bodybuilders and fitness experts maintain a strict diet that enhances the way they look and the way they build muscles, we must feed our brain the nutrients it needs.

It's not hard.

Here's an ideal day's menu.

We recommend you start the day by mixing a tablespoon of **flaxseeds** in with your breakfast – preferably a bowl of heart-healthy oatmeal.

Flaxseed contains an abundance of alpha-linolenic acid. It's a healthy fat that helps keep your cerebral cortex in good shape.

Almonds are another good option. Just a handful in the morning will help boost your memory and increase your attention span.

For lunch, it's no surprise we recommend a big salad. But make sure it contains ample **spinach** leaves and **lentils**.

Dark greens like spinach help slow the decline of our brain's function. Researchers at Chicago's Rush University tracked nearly 1,000 seniors over a five-year period.

They found that folks who ate just one or two servings of green leafy vegetables daily had the same mental sharpness as somebody 11 years younger.

Lentils are loaded with micronutrients that contribute to optimal brain function. Not to mention they're a great source of filling fiber, which helps lower cholesterol.

They're packed with protein – 18 grams in a one-cup serving – and help balance your body's pH level, promoting healthy gut bacteria.

That's huge.

For dinner, we recommend foods that are high in **omega-3 fatty acids**. The essential fatty acid not only is critical for heart health but also has shown itself to be a significant player in overall brain function.

Perhaps this is why we had so many powerful ideas while living in Alaska – our diet was rich with omega-3 stalwarts like **halibut** and **salmon**.

Other key dinnertime ingredients are **whole grains** like brown rice, barley, quinoa and couscous. They are high in fiber, complex carbohydrates and, once again, omega-3s.

But what's key about whole grains is they slowly release glucose into our brain... giving it a shot of long-lasting fuel.

And finally... dessert.

While few sugary treats can be considered healthy, there are some proven benefits to **dark chocolate**.

When it comes to brain health, our favorite form of candy is known for its ability to get our body to release dopamine – a chemical vital to brain function that's also important in learning and memory.

Fuel for Thought

Putting it all together, it's key to understand that mental decline due to aging doesn't occur because of the loss of brain cells.

No, it happens because the remaining cells become less efficient at communicating with one another.

Anything we can do to enhance the way our cells talk to each other goes a long way in boosting mental acuity.

The food we eat plays a huge role.

Give your brain a solid workout... but don't forget to fuel it with the good stuff.

Nature's Remedy for Heart Health

We have critical Know-How that will change the way you look at the food you eat.

It may even reduce your chances of a sudden heart attack.

We all know that salt is one of life's necessary evils. Too little of it and we die. Too much of it and our ticker tends to go haywire.

Docs have long known that too much sodium intake leads to things like high blood pressure and heart disease.

But what most folks don't understand is there's a mineral that acts in almost the exact opposite way.

The more of it you eat, the less effect salt will have on your body.

Nature's Remedy

In fact, the ratio of our salt intake to our potassium intake is one of the most important factors for our health... and yet virtually nobody talks about it.

Right now, the average American has a sodium-to-potassium ratio of 1.36-to-1.

That's not good.

A more "natural" diet – if we foraged for our food and didn't buy processed and preservative-loaded food from the grocery store – would have us eating 16 times as much potassium as sodium.

We're way out of whack.

The effects of our modern high-sodium diet are well-known.

The way our body deals with salt is quite simple.

Our kidneys act as the filters that get rid of excess salt. Most of the time, they can't keep up with our high-sodium diets. To combat the problem, our body holds on to water that works to dilute the salt.

But as this water builds up, it means our blood contains more fluid... and more fluid in our veins and arteries leads to, naturally, higher pressure within them.

It's no different from trying to cram more water into our garden hose. Pressure will rise.

Do it long enough or at high enough pressure and eventually something will wear out.

It's why high blood pressure leads to heart attacks, strokes and other serious cardiovascular issues.

Eat This, Not That

The best way to counteract this action – aside from popping another pill from Big Pharma – is to **maintain a healthy sodium-to-potassium ratio**.

That simply means cutting back on salt and ramping up our potassium intake.

The effects are clear.

A Harvard study showed that folks with the highest sodium intakes had a 20% higher risk of death than the folks on the opposite end of the scale. At the very same time, the folks who ranked highest for potassium intake had a 20% lower risk of dying than folks with less of this key mineral in their diet.

> ***Pair With Potassium:*** Lots of folks with high blood pressure take some sort of diuretic pill each day. But nature has her own cures, too. Take the **hibiscus plant**, for example. It's a natural diuretic, plus it prevents the body from getting rid of potassium. It's a good excuse to try some hibiscus tea.

It's not hard to maintain a healthy ratio.

Fresh fruits and vegetables, of course, are always a good bet. They contain very little salt and plenty of potassium.

But foods like **white beans**, **yogurt**, **potatoes** (white and sweet) and **salmon** top the list. **Spinach**, too, has nearly seven times as much potassium as it does salt.

On the other end of things, though, are the deadly processed foods.

A can of chicken soup, for instance, has six times as much salt as potassium. Meanwhile, a slice of pizza has an unhealthy ratio of nearly 4-to-1.

Avoid them.

It's that simple.

For good heart health, eat less salt and more potassium. It's a vital ratio... that could save your life.

How to Naturally Go With the Flow

Most men are confident with a joint knife. They've put up some drywall in their day – or, at the very least, patched a hole or two. Peeling paint on the garage? No sweat. Heck, when we're done, maybe we'll put up some new gutters.

Just please don't let it be the plumbing…

That's when the curse words start flying. Those ancient pipes behind our walls are hidden and rusty.

You've been there, hulking away under the sink, arms bent in ways you never thought possible. The root of the issue is obscured from view, and every moment you spend poking and prodding in the dark, there's a faint dripping sound to remind you that more damage is being done… somewhere.

It's why even the boldest of Mr. Fix-Its grimaces as he lifts his heavy-duty pipe wrench – the one that normally collects dust in the old tool chest.

He knows that all hell has broken loose… and failure is not an option.

Yet even as we reluctantly toil with the system that pumps life-giving water throughout our homes… many of us take for granted the system that gives life to our bodies and keeps our hearts beating. Out of sight, out of mind. *Until something goes wrong.*

For just as copper piping grows corroded and clogged with age... so do the veins inside of us. And the results – as impossible as it may seem to the waterlogged amateur plumber – can be even more calamitous.

Poor circulation doesn't just reduce the speed at which your body heals itself. It can squelch your sex drive, cause chronic pain and, oh yes, kill you.

Here are just a few of the deadly conditions that can arise when healthy blood cells have a tough time traveling through your body:

- High blood pressure
- Peripheral artery disease
- Stroke
- Kidney damage
- Aneurysm.

But it's your heart that assumes the most risk. Poor circulation is a big part of why, every 40 seconds in America, someone goes into cardiac arrest.

Cardiovascular diseases claim more lives than every form of cancer combined. They're responsible for 1 in 7 U.S. deaths. And a man's odds of experiencing a heart attack go up just as soon as he hits his 65th birthday.

The numbers are alarming, to be sure. Fortunately, there are some easy ways to avoid becoming another sad statistic.

In as little as a few weeks' time, even folks who currently suffer from poor circulation can unclog their internal plumbing.

It will just require some dietary changes and a bit of sweat. (But hey, at least there won't be any emergency trips to the hardware store.)

We'll start with what's easiest...

Eat This... Not That

It should come as no surprise that healthy circulation starts with a healthy diet. Of course, in the internet age, "healthy" is a relative term. So we must aim for foods that have a proven ability to improve circulation.

Our beloved **salmon** is a perfect example. Everyone knows that the hearty fish contains a generous amount of omega-3 fatty acids. Omega-3s have been proven to decrease triglyceride levels, slow the growth of atherosclerotic plaque, relieve joint pain and help lower blood pressure.

What you may not know is that salmon also contains natural blood-thinning properties and anticoagulants. That makes it a great – and delicious – way to tackle poor circulation. In fact, the American Heart Association (AHA) recommends you eat two servings per week.

Add some fresh, wild-caught salmon to your diet today.

And while you're at it...

Don't forget your fruits and veggies.

Kale – yes, the dreaded *kale* – is rich in chlorophyll. It's why the leaves of the crunchy greens are so... well, green. But the important thing to understand is that, on a molecular level, chlorophyll is quite similar to hemoglobin (the protein that moves oxygen through our bloodstream). Because of this, kale can help you quickly replenish your red blood cells.

Top your kale salad with some **beets**, and you'll *really* be cooking...

For decades, athletes have relied on beets as a natural way to improve stamina.

Studies have shown that the love-it-or-hate-it root vegetable can improve walking performance and reduce pain in patients with peripheral artery disease.

But the benefits of beets go far beyond athletics.

According to the AHA, "Nitrate consumption in the form of beet root juice can significantly elevate plasma nitrite levels that influence blood pressure and exercise tolerance." (Other root vegetables with circulation-boosting properties include ginger, maca and radishes.)

Vitamin C-rich fruits should also be a big part of your diet. Few folks realize it, but oranges and grapefruits are natural blood thinners. Pink grapefruits, in particular, contain a powerful antioxidant known as lycopene, which has been linked to improved circulation.

And while there aren't any official studies to confirm it, many experts believe citrus fruits can strengthen capillary walls. They may even prevent plaque buildup in your arteries.

Some other foods, spices and supplements to consider include...

- **Cayenne and chili pepper:** If you don't mind a little heat, these peppers (either raw or as dried spices) have proven to be good at fortifying blood vessels. Research shows they can also speed up your metabolism.

- **Ginkgo biloba**: Many seniors take this popular supplement to improve memory. But what you may not know is that ginkgo biloba stimulates better brain function by increasing blood flow throughout the body. It's a circulation booster for any age group.

- **Apricot, tomato and watermelon:** Like grapefruit, these fruits (lest we forget, the tomato is technically a fruit) get their reddish color from the powerful antioxidant lycopene. And if improving circulation isn't enough, researchers believe lycopene has cancer-fighting properties as well.

But keep in mind that a proper diet will take you only so far.

Be Like Teddy

The other half of our plan involves **exercise**. If you're an active person already, there probably isn't much you need to do. But if you're not, the advice here is simple... get moving.

The best exercises for improving circulation are those that engage your limbs. Working on a **punching bag**, for example, will get blood busily pumping through your arms and down to your feet. The punches don't need to be rapid. And they don't need to carry a ton of force. The main thing is to alternate your arms and control your breathing.

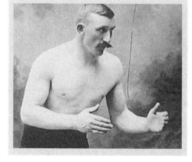

Push-ups are another great exercise. Again, we're looking to get the blood moving throughout our body. When done right, a push-up works at least five critical muscle groups: arms, chest, shoulders, abs and back. But remember, you're also balancing on your palms and feet. So, as a byproduct, you're engaging all four of your limbs as well.

Add three sets of 20 push-ups to your morning routine. You'll be amazed at how fast you start to feel – and see – the difference. Of course, not every circulation-boosting exercise must be extreme. **Going for brisk half-hour walks** will do wonders for your cardiovascular health. There's a reason why history is filled with great men who made walking part of their daily fitness routines. John Adams reportedly put 3 miles on his shoes each day. And Teddy Roosevelt started each morning with a 6-mile constitutional.

Ankle pumps are another easy way to get your blood flowing. Simply stand in one place and transfer your weight from the ball of one foot to the other. Alternate every couple of seconds. It won't take long for you to start to feel a little heat in your calf muscles. That's good; your calves are surrounded by some major veins and arteries. If you want to avoid painful clogs and clots, you'll want to get the blood flowing down there often.

Like we said, what's important is that you get moving. Our modern conveniences have made it easier than ever to be sedentary. And when you spend the whole day sitting, not only does it decrease your circulation... but the Centers for Disease Control and Prevention (CDC) warns you also have a higher risk of stroke, depression and certain types of cancer.

But if you combine an active lifestyle with the superfoods we mentioned earlier... you have the ultimate recipe for a healthy life.

Studies show you'll have more energy during the day... and you'll be calmer in your downtime.

Plus, your sex drive will be stronger... and the act itself more enjoyable.

As cardiologist Dean Ornish says, "Comprehensive changes in diet and lifestyle can improve blood flow not only to the heart, but to other organs as well." (And in case you're wondering... yes, the good doctor is hinting at *that organ*.)

Just take good care of your "plumbing." Remember... failure is not an option.

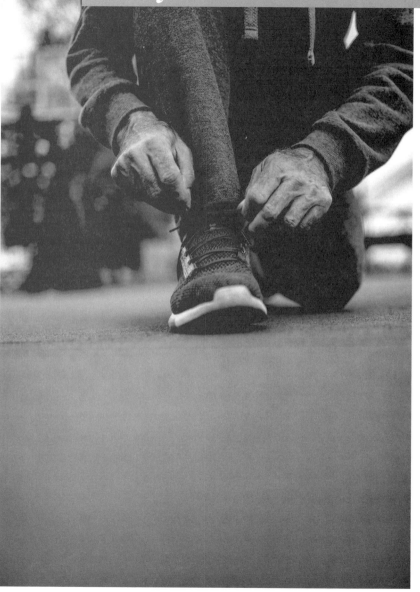

Exercise These Key Muscles to Get (and Stay) in Shape

Repeat... repeat... repeat... It's no secret that the more we do something, the better we get at it.

But what *is* secret is exactly why it works... and how you can use something we call "zombie muscles" to get in shape and stay that way.

When we first entered the law enforcement world, we drilled with our sidearms daily. Some of our fellow cadets griped about it. "Most of us will never even use our guns," they quipped, "and yet we train with them the most."

On the face of it, it's a fair argument.

Dig deeper, though, and it falls apart like a bad lie.

Training Our Brain

The truth is our muscles must rely on three key parts of the brain for nearly every complex movement. The motor cortex does the planning of the movement. The basal ganglia gets it going. And the cerebellum fixes things along the way that may not be quite right.

When we first ride a bike – or shoot a gun – all three parts of the brain must communicate and coordinate each precise movement. It's why most kids wobble and fall when they first hop on two wheels.

It's also why, with just a few hours of steady practice, they become steady and smooth, conquering hills without fear.

And as we all know, once those skills are mastered... they aren't forgotten.

It's why we spend hour after hour on the gun range. Few cops want to wait on their brains to figure out what to do when the bad guy is closing in. Their reactions must be natural and familiar – like hopping on a bike.

But there's new science out that tells us this ability to permanently learn a skill has much further-reaching implications than once believed.

It's all thanks to "zombie" muscles.

This is nuts.

> *"Zombie" Muscles*: The dormant nuclei in our muscle cells that help us to permanently learn a physical skill.

Sleeper Cells

There's a common belief that if we exercise regularly and suddenly stop that we'll soon start losing everything that we built. We fear that if a man gets big and strong, he'll lose it all if he stops exercising.

It's true that his muscle mass may slowly degrade... but he won't lose everything he built.

Far from it.

You see, in order to build muscle, our bodies do something quite miraculous. As we exercise, the cells that make up our muscles gain nuclei. Where most cells just have one nucleus, our muscles have the ability to have several of the DNA banks. And once a cell has created an extra nucleus, it doesn't easily give it up.

The nucleus simply lies dormant. It becomes a zombie muscle.

That's why when researchers at Ohio University recently put a group of women into a rigorous exercise program for 20 weeks and then let them lounge for eight months, their zombie muscles helped them to significantly outperform a group of women who had no prior exercise experience.

In other words, **exercise** has some previously unknown compound effects.

Even if we stop exercising today... our efforts will help us get back in shape later in our life.

That's good, but it's not the truly crazy news.

No, to get to that, we must understand the function of those extra DNA banks in our cells.

You see, a cell's nucleus serves as a sort of brain for each of our cells. It's the computer that decodes the messages in our DNA.

But there's research that shows many of the nuclei created by exercise have different components of our DNA switched on than our old DNA.

It's almost like creating a new body.

As new genes are turned on and others are turned off, the overall chemistry of our body changes.

It's why folks who start a long-term exercise plan quickly realize that their body simply acts differently... and it's almost always better.

And now thanks to this new research, we know that many of the changes may be permanent.

The takeaway from all of this is clear.

Yes, we should exercise more. That's a no-brainer. But we should also understand that once we build zombie muscles, they'll help us feel better and get more done long after we put the weights down.

Repeat... repeat... repeat.

Your Health Depends on Getting Up

We don't often align ourselves with Silicon Valley – in fact, usually we do *the exact opposite* – but when it comes to healthy living, we have to agree with Apple CEO Tim Cook...

Sitting, he says, is "the new cancer."

True, Cook made the statement as part of a pitch to sell smartwatches. (For as little as $249, Apple's signature timepiece will occasionally remind you to stand up.) But that fact aside, we applaud him for bringing this idea into the spotlight.

In a few centuries, we've gone from plowing fields and chasing down beasts to feed our families... to thumbing a few buttons and making sure to thank the delivery boy.

Unfortunately, our bodies haven't caught up to all of our modern conveniences.

And if you fall into the same comfy trap as so many others... the results could be deadly.

Hardly Healthy Living

Fact is, there are heaps of evidence that show just how dangerous a sedentary lifestyle can be.

The CDC warns that inactive adults have a higher risk of heart disease, stroke and depression.

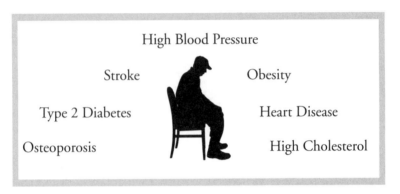

According to one study, folks who spend most of their day sitting have up to a 66% higher risk of developing certain types of cancer.

Another study found a link between sedentary behavior and Type 2 diabetes risk.

And yet another suggests that sitting for prolonged periods of time can lead to decreased brain function.

Obviously we're big proponents of staying active. We don't just *write* essays on fixing our cars, tending to our bees and tromping through the forest... we practice what we preach.

But in our modern society, we're quickly becoming exceptions to the rule.

After a long day in front of the computer, most office workers – and most retirees – spend their evenings glued to the boob tube. They catch up on the latest "viral sensation" from Netflix while scrolling mindlessly through social media feeds.

"I need to unplug," they say... as they plug in.

It's hardly healthy living.

And as we said, this behavior is downright dangerous.

But you *can* beat it.

A Simple Health Tip to Prolong Your Life

Researchers have found that if you sit for more than eight hours a day, you must engage in at least **one hour of moderate to vigorous exercise** to counteract all the damage your cushy desk chair is doing to your body.

Go for a brisk walk... do some push-ups... just do *something*.

And don't stop there...

According to Dr. Marc Hamilton, director of the Texas Obesity Research Center, "Sitting too much is not the same as exercising too little."

His health tip? Instead of getting in one substantial workout then loafing around, you should aim to get steady light exercise throughout the day.

Or, even better, do both. That is, kick off your morning with some intensive exercise and make sure to keep moving in the hours that follow.

"Exercise is good for you for one reason," says Hamilton, "but light activity is good for you for another reason... you can't assume that one will replace the other."

Life is filled with distractions. At the end of a long day, it's easy to justify plopping down on the couch and staring mindlessly at a screen. But that's an urge you must fight.

Research has proven... your health depends on it.

And if research doesn't motivate you, take it from Walt Whitman:

> *To you, clerk, literary man, sedentary person, man of fortune, idler... Up!*
>
> *The world (perhaps now you look upon it with pallid and disgusted eyes) is full of zest and beauty for you, if you approach it in the right spirit!*

Make This Part of Your Daily Routine

Walking is one of the best exercises... not only for our bodies, but for our minds.

We know the weight-shedding benefits of walking.

There's nothing new on that front...Going by some rough math – the numbers vary depending on your speed, weight and terrain – we can expect to burn about 200 calories for every 30 minutes of walking. With no other changes to our diet or daily routine, that moderate amount of exercise will cut about two pounds off our body in a month.

It won't qualify us for any "before and after" pictures, but it's a whole lot better than sitting on the couch.

And the health effects aren't all focused on losing weight.

Medicine for Your Brain

According to the fine folks at Harvard, a brisk walk each day boosts our immune system.

Of the 1,000 walkers they tracked who walked at least 20 minutes daily for five days each week, 43% of them had fewer sick days than folks who walked one day or less.

And the American Cancer Society found that women who walked seven or more hours each week had a 14% lower chance of developing breast cancer than those who walked half that time.

And get this... there's now research that shows walking may help stave off Alzheimer's disease. A study led by a doctor at the University of Pittsburgh found that a test group that walked briskly for 40 minutes three days each week increased the volume of their hippocampus – a critical area of the brain that is key to our memory and which is ravaged by Alzheimer's disease.

It's all because a few things happen in our bodies when we walk.

First, the obvious... our heart beats faster. As it does, our brain gets more blood and therefore more oxygen. The better fueled this critical organ, the better it works – and, as we'll see in a minute, the better we think.

Also, a protein called brain-derived neurotrophic factor is released as we walk. It's a bit complicated, but this ultra-important chemical helps protect our most vital organ and, importantly, helps to repair our memory neurons.

Scientists often refer to it as a sort of chemical reset switch.

Mind Games

Perhaps most interesting, though, is the startling connection between a daily stroll and our thoughts.

It helps explain why some of the most successful men in American history were devoted walkers.

"How vain it is to sit down to write when you have not stood up to live!" Henry David Thoreau once wrote in his journal. "Methinks that the moment my legs begin to move, my thoughts begin to flow."

Many writers make walking part of their normal creative routines. And now we have scientific proof of why it works.

A couple of researchers at Stanford recently showed yet again that walking significantly boosts our creativity.

They asked a group of 176 college students to do imaginative tasks like thinking of unusual uses for ordinary objects. The students who were told to walk and think, on average, thought of between four and six more unique uses than those who were sitting.

Study after study shows similar results. It's fascinating.

Bottom line... if you want to be creative, get on your feet.

A Time and Place

But where you walk matters. The reason this simple exercise is so profoundly good for our mind is because it's quite simple for us to do. It gets the heart flowing and increases the oxygen in our brain without the need for us to concentrate on the physical movement.

That's why walking in simple, pastoral settings is best.

Thoreau had it right. Get out of the city and into the woods.

Any natural setting works just fine. Most researchers agree, though, that having water nearby is ideal. The sounds and simple imagery allow our minds to wander to fresh and new things... without the distraction of unnatural noises or cluttered city streets.

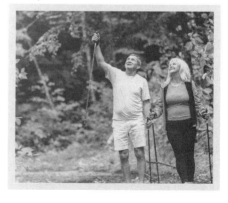

And while any time is a good time for a walk, early has proven to be the best time. It gets your mind flowing and ready for the day ahead.

If you're looking for a simple, enjoyable activity that will help you lose weight, stave off deadly diseases and think better... walking is it.

A Simple Exercise to Combat a Life-Threatening Disorder

A local school recently asked us to talk with its students. Even with a busy schedule, there was no way we could refuse.

The timing was perfect.

Just as we scratched our head wondering how in the world we'd connect with these kids (should we talk about the evils of Big Government... discuss the War on Men... or perhaps teach them how to pick a good stock?), the mainstream press caught on to what we've been shouting for quite a while now... that cellphones are killing our kids.

As usual, it wasn't reason or morality that got the press' attention.

It was money.

In case you missed it, two huge investors in Apple griped quite loudly about the devastating impact of cellphones on kids. They cited studies. They showed the nasty effects teachers are seeing. And they poked a finger at the oh-so-young age at which kids are getting phones these days.

With those winds at our back, we took to the stage.

We talked of our background living off the grid, the power of disconnecting from the electronic world and the utter importance of what we dub a healthy dose of "**vitamin O**" – **the great outdoors**.

We knew we hit the right message when folks in the audience begged us to give the same message to their groups.

But the truth is what's happening today isn't just affecting kids.

No, it's devastating the lives of millions of Americans...

Where'd They Go?

It's not something we write about all that often, but the nasty health effects of our electronic culture are a topic we can't ignore.

Anytime we discuss the subject, we point to a big, scary number.

Each year, some 152 million Americans don't go outside for recreation.

That's *half of our nation* not doing what a full 100% of our country was forced to do just a few generations ago.

It's no wonder obesity, diabetes and even depression are on the rise.

The data show outdoor participation peaked roughly a generation ago. After steadily increasing for more than 50 years, the number of folks getting outdoors started to decline somewhere between 1981 and 1991.

Now it's falling at a clip of roughly 1% each year.

There's a clear correlation between the numbers.

The less time we spend outdoors, the sicker we get.

Folks in the know call it *nature deficit disorder*.

It's affecting our kids in a big way.

Instead of letting them experience the healing power of ol' Ma Nature, we'd rather push some pills down their throats and tell them how dangerous it is out there.

But it's also hurting those of us who may have fewer hairs on our heads these days.

Many experts, in fact, say the problem is so large – and the effects of getting outdoors so great – that we could be looking at the first generation that has a shorter life span than their parents.

> ***Nature deficit disorder:*** The less time we spend outdoors, the sicker we get.

That's crazy.

Especially when you consider the fact that "contracting" nature deficit disorder is *entirely avoidable*.

A Dose of Vitamin O Leads to Better Health

The health effects of getting outdoors are well-known.

For instance, science has proven that folks who spend more time outside recover from injuries faster. The exposure to natural light plays a significant role in how our bodies heal.

In fact, the amount of vitamin D in our bodies is directly related to the amount of time we spend in the sun. Just 15 minutes each day can lead to better health. It's been proven to boost our immune system and help us achieve a more positive outlook.

Being outdoors also boosts energy levels.

Living in Alaska, we'd often take folks on long, scenic hikes. They'd start out moaning about how tired they were. And yet they'd readily admit they were full of energy by the time we finished the hike.

They'd also note an increase in focus and creativity.

It's no wonder some of the most influential leaders in American history made a walk an obligatory part of their daily routine. John Adams, as I mentioned, trekked at least 3 miles each day... at the age of 77.

But the research shows it doesn't take an endurance hike to get the benefits of being outside. No, better health can start with a simple 20-minute walk through the woods. Even a quick jaunt through a lush park each day will get the job done.

That's why the next time we talk to a bunch of kids, we're not doing it from a stage. Nope, we're headed outside and off on a hike.

It may just save a life.

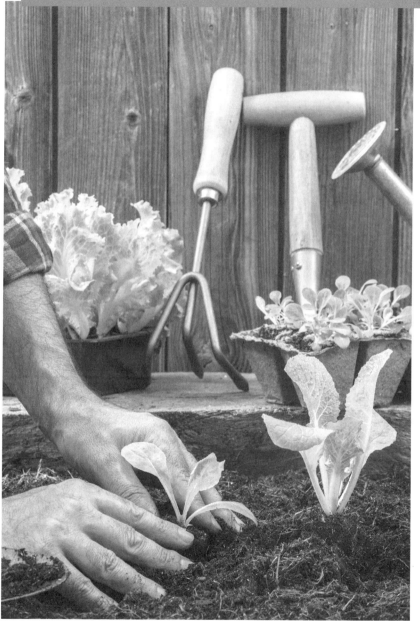

Sustainable Living Starts Here

We have a profound question for you. Is the land that surrounds you "nurturing"?

The question came up during a conversation with an off-the-grid architect. It's a vital question worth far more than the few hundred words that will follow.

Asking it leads us to a key idea we all must understand...Belize is a unique country. I've spent some time in a small, poor town tucked quite close to the Guatemalan border.

Most homes there seem to sprout right from the fertile land. There are gardens in the backyard, chickens in the front and likely a steer roaming somewhere nearby.

It's no wonder the region is quickly becoming the heart of the off-the-grid community.

The land nurtures.

Survival or Sustainable Living?

Our architect friend summed it up well. "You can stockpile all the canned foods you want," he said. "But eventually you'll run out. That's when you'll pray your land can take care of you."

With that idea in mind, let's ask our question at the top a different way.

Could you live off your land?

If you live in a city or anything less than a rural situation, you're worried. There's no way you could live off the land, right?

Well, actually, anybody can do it... no matter where they live. I'll explain in a minute.

I'm lucky. Our microfarm could sustain our family endlessly.

It's 30 acres, but the layout was thoughtful and the land is fertile. Between the garden, pasture and apiary, we've got more than enough meat, vegetables and honey.

But, again, our location was planned with sustainable living in mind.

We live in the country, surrounded by farms and forests. Most folks don't.

Some 81% of Americans live in a city or in the suburbs. Hauling pigs through your cul-de-sac isn't conducive to keeping happy neighbors.

But that's okay. You don't need to live on your "nurturing" land.

You only need access to it.

The Ultimate Connection

There's an underground movement slowly gaining momentum in the United States.

Once the realm of hippies and Subaru-driving granola eaters, community gardens are becoming quite popular... even with the antisocial prepper crowd.

It makes perfect sense.

Gardening and farming are becoming a lost art... a lost art that could also keep you alive.

There once was a time when the vast majority of men could live off the land. They likely grew up on a farm and never had to "learn" vital survival skills. That knowledge was part of normal, everyday life.

Those days are over.

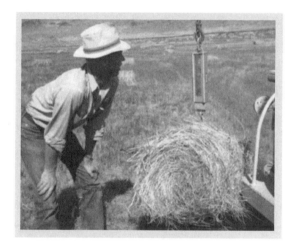

Most men these days have never felt the delight of going from seed to bounty. They've rarely visited a farm, let alone lived on one.

But community gardens offer the solution.

They're sprouting up across the nation. New York, Detroit, Baltimore, Los Angeles... they all have vibrant community gardens.

It's a noble trend. For just a few bucks a year, you can rent a plot. It's yours to do what you want with.

Grow peas... beans... hot peppers... whatever.

If you're a homebrewer, try it out and grow some of your own hops. A small 20-by-20-foot plot could sustain a family of four if managed correctly.

Just grow something. Learn the art. Get connected with your land. Let it nurture you.

You'll gain knowledge, live a healthier, more relaxed life and have a reliable supply of food.

Our connection to the land is ultimately what sustains us. Whether it's a survival situation after a major catastrophe... whether we're living off the grid like our friends in Belize... or whether we simply want to live richer, more fulfilled lives. Focus on a nurturing connection with the land.

It's the ultimate connection.

How to Grow a Sustainable Crop of Healthy Food Indoors

Interest in urban farming has soared in recent years. A lot of the attention, rightfully, seems to be coming from folks curious about the "prepper" lifestyle. Others are attracted to the idea of off-the-grid living and building their own tiny homestead farm.

But one fact is indisputable... *Being able to grow a sustainable crop of healthy food is Know-How every man should have.*

In 1960, more than 30% of the population lived in a rural setting. Today, that percentage has fallen into the teens. Modern men have no idea how to raise their own chickens or tend to crops. Instead...

We rely on big-box retailers to provide nourishment for our families... We eat mass-produced, hormone-injected meats... And we consume fruits and vegetables coated in harmful chemicals.

Whether you're interested in urban farming as a hobby or taking a deep dive into the homesteading or off-the-grid lifestyle, it's imperative that you know how to grow your own healthy food.

And with the simple (and cheap) DIY hydroponic system we lay out below, you can do exactly that...

The Ultimate Urban Farming Setup

In case you're unfamiliar with the concept, hydroponic farming is a way to grow plants without soil. As the "hydro" in the name suggests, this is most often done in water.

The advantages of hydroponic farming over traditional farming are numerous. For one thing, you can grow anywhere: indoors, outdoors... even *vertically*. Because of this, hydroponic gardens yield more crops in less space. Even better, those crops <u>require only 10% of the water</u> soaked up by field-grown plants.

There are lots of ways to get into the world of hydroponic farming. But we consider our setup the ultimate "starter kit" because it A) is cheap, B) is easy to assemble and C) works.

With tools and materials in hand, you should be up and running in less than an hour's time.

But before we get into specifics, an important note about lighting...

Three Lighting Options (And Our Personal Favorite)

When it comes to lighting, you have several choices.

Some serious growers prefer high-intensity discharge (HID) grow lights, which use lots of electricity and generate a ton of heat. (The upside is that HIDs are powerful enough to grow a full range of produce, from leafy greens to hearty vegetables.)

Or you could go with fluorescent lighting, which is cheaper to run but sufficient only if you're growing lettuce or herbs.

In our view, LED is the way to go. You'll pay more initially (approximately $100 to $150), but an LED grow lamp can provide adequate lighting to support everything from baby spinach to watermelon. Plus, LED bulbs are far gentler on your energy bill.

The trick is to buy a grow lamp that contains both red and blue bulbs. That way you can plant virtually any crop you want.

You should be able to find all three of these options at your local hardware store or garden center.

And when all else fails, there's always Amazon.

Once you've secured your lighting rig – easily the most expensive part of the whole operation – you can get to building the main part of our hydroponic farming system.

And if you're thrifty, the rest of the materials should cost you **less than 10 bucks**.

Here's what you'll need:

- Aquarium bubbler/air pump
- Aquarium tubing (should come with bubbler)
- Net cups
- Rockwool cubes (aka "starter plugs")
- And a 1-gallon (or larger) plastic pail <u>with a lid</u>.

You'll also need a drill and an appropriately sized bit to make holes in the pail lid. The exact size will depend on the width of the net cups you'll be using (and what you're growing). For our purposes, we're going to assume you're using 2-inch net cups and, thus, a 2-inch hole saw bit.

To get started, make evenly spaced 2-inch holes in the pail lid, along with one smaller hole for the aquarium tubing to feed through.

With holes made (and debris cleared), you'll want to set your bubbler in the pail.

Run the tubing up the side of the pail and out the small hole you made. This will allow for aeration, which is vital to healthy nutrient circulation. (As an added bonus, aeration in a hydroponic system helps your seedlings grow much faster than if they were planted in soil.)

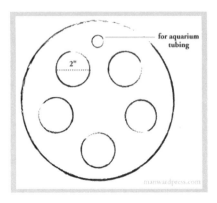

Next, fill the pail with water. The water should be practically touching the lid (you'll see why in a moment).

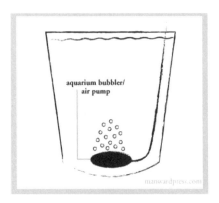

With that all done, it's time to focus on your actual plants...

First things first: Soak the rockwool cubes – one for each 2-inch hole you drilled – in water for at least one hour.

Once your rockwool is good and soaked, it's time to add your seeds. Push a couple into the center of each cube. Then set the cubes into the net cups.

Place the net cups into the 2-inch holes you drilled in the pail lid.

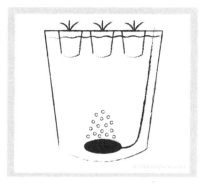

Now plug in your bubbler, set the entire system underneath the lighting rig you picked out and boom... there you have it.

You've just built your own indoor hydroponic garden.

Rockwool: What It Is and Where to Find It

Rockwool cubes – also known as stonewool cubes or grow blocks – are composed of spun-together mineral fibers. They're great for sucking up water, air and important nutrients, which are then pulled into your plant's roots.

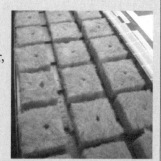

Garden centers and online retailers sell rockwool cubes by the sheet.

As of this writing, you can buy a sheet of 200 cubes on Amazon for less than $0.10 per cube.

Depending on the types of plants you start with, seedlings should emerge within a matter of days.

You'll be harvesting your first crop of organic, healthy food in just a few weeks' time.

It's the perfect urban farming setup for folks who want to be prepared but lack the outdoor space to grow their own fruits, vegetables and herbs.

And even if you have room on your property for an ample-sized garden, growing food indoors can give you some added peace of mind.

The Simple (Must-Know) Food Trick Could Save Your Life

It was one of the most important inventions of the 19th century. It saved lives and reshaped the world. It helped win wars, and it spawned millionaires.

What's crazy is you can now do it in your own kitchen.

Canning changed countless lives... and it could save yours.

The ability to store foods for long periods of time meant man could explore further, fight harder and share foods from around the world.

Canning changed the way the world eats. It brought salmon south from Alaska. It turned lobster into a rich man's food. And it allows us to store months' or even years' worth of food in our pantry... without the need for refrigeration or preservatives.

Easy... and Easier

The technique of heating food beyond the boiling point and then sealing it in an airtight container was invented by Nicolas Appert. He did it in response to a call from Napoleon, who was desperate for a way to feed his hungry armies spreading throughout Europe.

The idea is quite simple... which is why it's an ideal skill to learn.

There are two primary ways to preserve food through canning: the boiling water bath method and pressure canning.

Pressure canning takes special equipment, but it's the only safe way to preserve meat and seafood. With this technique, jars of food are placed in water, which is heated to more than 240 degrees (the high temperature kills the spores responsible for botulism).

Because the water must exceed its boiling point, special equipment is needed. It's not all that expensive, though. You can find a suitable pressure canner for less than a hundred bucks online... less if you buy a used one locally.

If you're just canning tomatoes, fruits and jellies, though, you can use the simpler water bath method.

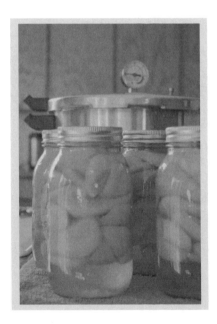

In this case, simply place the filled and sealed jars in boiling water for the prescribed amount of time (each type of food differs). Once removed from the heat, the air inside the jar cools, shrinks and forms an airtight vacuum in the container.

The food is good for at least a year.

Good Eatin'

What's interesting about canning is that it locks in the nutritional value of food.

Unlike fresh fruits or vegetables that begin losing their nutritional value nearly immediately, canned foods hold on to their vitamins.

In fact, recent research shows that some foods (like pumpkin) actually see a spike in nutrients when canned.

Even better, canning gives you food that is free from harmful preservatives and additives.

Canning – no matter which technique you choose – is an ideal way to store excess food.

A Lost Art... That You Can Eat

I t's good to be a carnivore. Come near our microfarm in the late fall and you'll surely catch a whiff of the sweet, inviting smell of wood smoke. Just a whiff of the hickory roasting in the bottom of our smoker tends to make the neighbors grab their forks and knock at the back door.

They love us this time of year.

We're **curing bacon**.

The recipe is simple: curing salt, kosher salt, a few tablespoons of brown sugar and, if we're feeling adventurous, some maple syrup or perhaps some honey from our hives.

From there, we rub the mix into the pork belly (that's the part with the nipples, if you're curious) and stuff it into the bottom shelf of the fridge for a week.

Once it turns the right shade of pink and the meat gets to the stiffness of a well-done steak (it'll have about the same give as the point of your chin), we'll wash it off, dry it a bit and toss it on the smoker for a few hours.

Bam... bacon like you can't find anywhere else.

We often forget the simplicity of the process.

After all, most folks are convinced the only way to get DIY bacon is to own a factory. They hear the (truthful) tales of slabs of pig getting poked by hundreds of needles filled with potentially cancerous preservatives and smoke flavoring and think there's no way they can make the stuff in their own kitchen.

Ancient and Simple

Bacon is perhaps the simplest form of cured meat. But no curing process is all that complicated. After all, our ancestors have considered it a vital skill for thousands of years.

Salted meat was part of the Mesopotamian diet as early as 3000 B.C.

Nearly 3,000 years later, the Romans were curing their pork.

And by A.D. 1000, the salt trade had become one of the most important economic functions on the planet.

But this primitive charcuterie wasn't about flavor or a chef's artistic expression. Far from it.

It was all about saving what we have today for tomorrow.

Knowing that lean times always lie ahead, the humans who ruled the land before us quickly learned how to preserve today's catch for tomorrow.

As they did, they were able to explore the world, survive harsh winters and even enter foreign trade.

No doubt the ability to cure meat changed the world.

And yet, modern man is virtually ignorant on the subject. This long-standing skill is all but dead today.

Cured meat these days is something most folks blindly buy at the grocery store.

Increasingly, it's becoming a specialty item that comes with a premium price tag. We've seen cured meat samplers – filled with meats that were once everyday items – selling for a hundred dollars or more.

With this simple skill, you can save those dollars and reap all the benefits.

With a quality piece of organic or grass-fed meat, you can enjoy (always in moderation) an irresistible treat packed with protein, B vitamins, an array of minerals and heart-healthy oleic acid.

Don't Just Eat This Miracle Food... Make It

Beekeeping is becoming a lost art. When I began my quest, all I wanted was some honey. I read a book about it, and it sounded interesting.

It's not hyperbole to say learning the skill changed my life.

Honey truly is a miracle food.

Honey is nature's best sweetener. It consists of about 69% glucose and fructose.

But unlike the processed sugar that's found loaded into so much of our food, honey is quite easy for your body to turn into useful energy.

It helps eliminate the energy peaks and valleys associated with store-bought white sugar.

Even better, it aids in weight loss.

The honey I grow on our microfarm is 100% organic and unprocessed.

There are no chemicals. It's not pasteurized. It's not even filtered.

The bees make it, and all I do is put it in jars.

Unrefined Is Just Fine

By far, raw honey is the best stuff.

But the health effects of honey are only one reason every man must know how to raise bees.

One of the greatest aspects of honey is that it doesn't spoil. Put a jar in your "go" bag and never worry about it expiring.

It can be added to crackers or homemade bread to provide a much-needed energy source.

This past year, I harvested 8 gallons of honey from two hives. If the need would arise, our pantry could keep us alive for months. By upping my production to five hives, I could expect about 20 gallons.

We keep the honey we need and sell the rest. If your goal is to raise bees as an income source, expect to break even in about two years.

It's not cheap to start harvesting honey.

But by sticking to the basics, you can start two hives (I always recommend starting with at least two hives) for about $450.

You'll need to order your bees and build or buy some hive boxes.

Plus, you'll need some essential beekeeping equipment.

But here's what most folks don't know about raising bees.

You can do it anywhere.

Simple Is Better

Most folks I talk to say they can't raise bees because they live in the city or in a subdivision.

They're wrong... urban beekeeping is quite popular. Done right, even your closest neighbors won't know you have bees.

And even if you can't raise bees at home, there's nothing stopping you from raising them on somebody else's land.

Most farmers will gladly let you put hives on their land. Most often, all they want in return is a quart or two of honey. It's cheap rent.

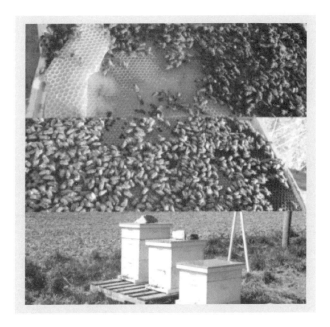

The hardest part of beekeeping is getting started. It sounds like a daunting, painful endeavor.

It's not.

Really, it's quite simple.

Like I said, for a few hundred bucks, you can get the boxes, frames, tools and enough bees to be harvesting honey within a year.

Start by watching a few videos, then read a book or two.

From there, find a local bee club and get started.

Beekeeping will teach you patience. It will create a source of income. It will humble you. And it will provide one of the healthiest foods on the planet.

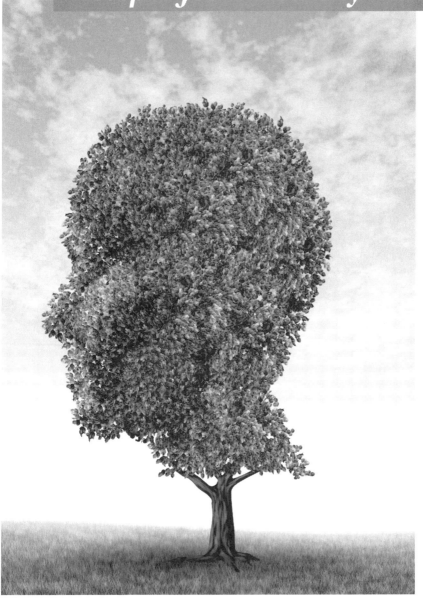

Part IV: Natural Recipes for a Healthy Mind

The Perfect Nighttime Ritual for Better, Restorative Sleep

W e've all been there. It's miserable. There are few things as frustrating as lying in bed at night and not being able to sleep.

We used to do it a lot... but then we uncovered a totally natural cure.

Rock bottom for us was lying in bed, wide awake until 2:30 in the morning worrying about just one dumb thing somebody said to us earlier.

Compounding the pain was the fact that we had a cross-country flight at 7:30 a.m.

It was misery.

We were determined to figure out how to sleep better. We vowed to find a cure.

We did. And it's oh-so-simple. Anybody can do it.

Like so many things, this cure takes us back to basics.

There's no modern technology... no pills... no gimmicks... just a good ol' fashioned **nightly ritual**.

About That Nightcap

The routine starts well before it's time to climb under the covers.

Most folks get this vital first step wrong. We're told a drink or two is good for us. It keeps the ticker tickin', they say.

Maybe so, but a recent review of 27 studies showed that just a single serving of alcohol can wreck a good night of sleep.

It's all about sleep patterns... particularly slow-wave patterns called delta activity. Alcohol inhibits this critical memory-forming type of deep sleep.

Plus, alcohol blocks the restoring effects of REM sleep – the sort of sleep that allows us to dream.

When we're robbed of this stage of slumber – even after eight hours in the sack – we're drowsy and have a hard time concentrating the next day.

If you want to sleep well, don't get duped into thinking booze is the cure.

Sure, it may help us get to sleep faster... but it's a dirty trick. We will not get a quality night of sleep.

If you really need something to drink, have a hot cup of (naturally decaffeinated) chamomile tea.

Our Enemy Strikes Again

Okay... so no booze. Got it.

Most folks have no problem skipping a drink. They'll get their dopamine fix from the 21st century's newest addiction... our archnemesis, the cellphone.

This is bad.

The research is quite clear.

Checking your phone or playing on your laptop before bed is one of the absolute worst things you can do.

You might as well have a cup of coffee.

A recent study by the National Sleep Foundation showed how bad this screen plague has become. A full 95% of folks surveyed admitted to using some sort of electronic device within an hour of going to bed.

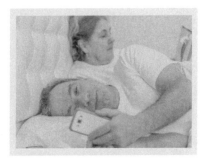

That's bad.

It undoubtedly plays a leading role in why some two-thirds of folks say they don't get enough sleep.

The problem is – according to the folks at Harvard Medical School – exposure to artificial light before bed suppresses the release of melatonin, the hormone that is critical to triggering sleep.

Plus, an onslaught of social media, news and, worse, text messages adds a layer of stress and thought that puts us in a mindset that is completely opposite of where we need to be when we climb in bed.

If you don't have the guts to throw your deadly cellphone away... at least **keep the phone out of the bedroom**.

How to Sleep Better

Instead of relaxing with a drink and a bit of web surfing – guilty? – do this simple old-timey exercise.

Ben Franklin is most famous for championing it, but our research has uncovered countless other great (and highly productive) folks who followed the same evening ritual.

First, set your schedule and keep to it.

Know exactly what time you are going to bed. Franklin hit the sack every night at 10:00 p.m. He got up at 5:00 a.m.

Pick a time and don't waver. Your body will soon know that when the time arrives, it's time to call it a day.

It sounds counterintuitive, but set an alarm to remind you when to go to bed.

That's what we did in the woods of Alaska when it was easy to hike until midnight in the perpetual sun of summer.

Franklin also wound down each night by reviewing his day. We've found this to be critical.

The Founding Father asked himself a key question... "What good have I done today?"

It's an ideal question to ask. It leads to self-reflection and adds a sense of accomplishment to our end-of-day routine.

But there are other questions that may suit your goals better.

"What were my three wins today?"

"What went well?"

"What am I most proud of?"

It's imperative that we keep our bedtime thoughts positive.

Our last thoughts of the day are not when we should focus on what we didn't get done or who made us mad. We must use them to reset our minds for the day to come.

Really, our ideal routine is quite simple.

Keep it quiet... keep it natural... and keep it basic.

How to Dramatically Improve Your Memory

F or some odd reason, we can remember where we went on summer vacation when we were just 6 years old... but we can't remember where in the world we put our keys last night.

It's no secret that as we age, our ability to remember things tends to diminish.

But it doesn't have to be this way.

Our minds are incredibly powerful... if we know how to use them properly.

Like hidden features in a new car, there are some simple tricks that help us get the most from our brain's built-in "accessories." But since our bodies don't yet come with a user's manual, most folks have no idea these tricks exist.

Remember This

It's the short-term memory that causes so many folks problems. It's quite lousy at its job.

The classical belief is that we can retain just five to nine pieces of information in our short-term memory at one time. But more recent research puts that figure even lower... at no more than four things.

That's why we can't remember if we took our pills this morning. It's because we're also trying to remember our keys... our grocery list... and the myriad tasks in the day ahead.

But our long-term memory bank is much, much richer. It's a whole different story.

Get this... Paul Reber, a psychologist at Northwestern University, thinks the brain can store an incredible 2.5 million gigabytes of information in the form of long-term memory. That's enough to download some 300 years' worth of TV.

If only we could tap that oh-so-deep well whenever we wanted.

Ah, but we can.

The Samos Mind Trick: A Quick (and Classic) Way to Improve Memory

This impressive memory trick isn't new. It's not the latest discovery from Harvard. And it doesn't require any modern "chemistry" from Big Pharma.

No, it's thousands of years old. And it's simple.

In fact, it was first used more than 2,500 years ago... by the same man who taught us how to measure the sides of a right triangle.

That's right, the same man who gave us the Pythagorean theorem – the man from Samos – can also teach us a thing or two about our brains and our memory.

Unlike today, back in the day of the great Greek philosophers and mathematicians, a man's memory was his most coveted faculty.

That's because they didn't have easy access to books or the internet (the worst memory killer of all). No, all they had was their brain.

A thinker like Pythagoras took his brain and its memory quite seriously.

That's why he did something peculiar every night before bed. He reviewed his entire day before he fell asleep for the night.

He didn't focus just on the big stuff or the need-to-know memories. He mentally recalled everything he did and learned from the second he got out of bed to the instant he crawled back in... *everything*.

It trained his mind to pay attention... It tapped that oh-so-powerful storage device between his ears.

For proof, Pythagoras would often recall a day's events weeks or even months after they happened. It was as if he were able to mentally record every second of his day.

Simple Trick... Big Benefits

You can – and should – do it, too.

It's a simple trick with many benefits. And it's not hard to do. We've already explained everything you need to know.

Simply get into bed each night and do your very best to recall the day's events – from start to finish. Focus on as much detail as possible. Work to recall numbers, colors, your thoughts... everything.

Do it in the order it happened. Don't skip around.

It will be quite tough at first. You'll recall just a fraction of the day's events. But soon – likely in just a few weeks – you'll be recalling huge chunks of data.

What's neat about this trick is the benefits stretch beyond your memory.

Sure, you'll be able to recall much more about your waking hours. (The days of forgetting your pills or losing your keys are over.) But you'll also find yourself doing things throughout the day to help boost your memory.

Some folks say this bedtime ritual helps them live more in the moment. They're much more aware of their day and how they spend their time.

Interestingly, an overlooked but important side effect of the technique is that it leads to better sleep. By focusing on the events of the day, our brain slowly relaxes and our thoughts lull us to sleep.

In fact, at first, you'll find that you fall asleep long before you remember the day's full events. That's okay. It's part of the process. Don't get frustrated. And certainly don't quit the exercise if you aren't able to recall an entire day at first.

With practice, you will.

You'll soon become a master of your memory.

Three Tricks to Change Your Mind

I'm going to play a bit of a mind game on you. Don't worry; it won't hurt. But the effects may be permanent.

I'm going to tell you something that is contrary to what you believe. I'll prove that what I'm telling you is 100% right. The evidence will be convincing... but you will still have great doubt.

The effort will highlight a dangerous flaw that lives in all of us.

But there is a solution – a solution that has the potential to greatly improve your life.

Here's the truth that you won't believe: Carrots don't do a thing for your vision.

Stick with me.

You see, I'm a man of habit. I eat several carrots every day on my way to the office. Nearly every time I tell someone of my habit, they comment with something like "Your night vision must be great."

This thing about carrots and vision is an idea that nearly all of us believe.

But the truth is the connection between the vegetable and its ability to boost our eyesight is pure bunk.

In fact – this is where it gets really tough to believe – the idea is pure government propaganda. It's a lie that was first perpetrated during World War II.

You've Been Duped

You see, the British government was the first to use onboard radar to detect enemy planes. No matter how dark it was outside, the Royal Air Force pilots were able to spot incoming planes on their displays and shoot them down.

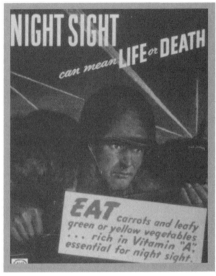

To the bad guys, it was magic. They had no idea how the Brits could see their planes sneaking through the nighttime sky.

But to the British, it was war-winning technology. They didn't want to give up their technology. So they lied.

They created a campaign that linked eating carrots with better vision.

It was pure junk science... but it worked. The Brits believed it. The Germans believed it. And amazingly, we still believe the lie some 75 years later.

But why?

Why is it that mankind can be so smart and yet so darn dumb?

The truth is a couple of phenomena are at work.

Are We That Dumb?

In a study published in the *Journal of Personality and Social Psychology* in 1993, researchers helped solve a 400-year-old debate about why we believe what we do.

Through a series of tests, the scientists clearly showed that humans nearly instantly believe what they are first told.

From there, it's up to further evidence and contemplation – something our lazy brains are rarely fond of – to **change our minds**.

It's great news for politicians and marketers... and very bad news for our pal the truth.

But the problem is compounded by another nasty human trait known as the confirmation bias – the tendency for us to stick to our initial beliefs by believing only evidence in their favor.

This trait is dangerous.

Despite all sorts of evidence and all sorts of campaigns, we believe what we're first taught.

It's a phenomenon that affects our everyday lives in many ways.

One deadly way this trait manifests is in the realm of our health.

It's why it took more than two generations for folks to believe smoking can kill us. It's why so many folks don't see the dangers in social media. And it's why, despite strong evidence to the contrary, many folks are ignorant of the cancer-causing effects of cellphone radiation.

Instead of believing new facts as they emerge... we believe what we're first told.

But this trait also affects our relationships.

It's a big reason we hold grudges and don't trust others. It's the reason our political stances rarely change.

And it's the reason fake news has managed to infiltrate our lives.

Beating Your Brain

Overcoming this nasty trait isn't all that difficult.

But first – ah, a Catch-22 – you must believe that confirmation bias is affecting your thoughts.

You must believe that what you first understand to be the truth may be wrong. And more important, you need to believe that your lazy survival-focused brain will do everything it can to keep you from changing your mind.

The confirmation bias is strong.

Use these three tricks to beat it:

- First, train yourself to understand that what you first believe is not necessarily right or wrong. It's likely somewhere in the middle. Embrace that idea and be eager and excited to discover the truth.

- Second, as you work to discover the truth, create three distinct hypotheses. Tracking three distinct ideas is important as it forces you to go beyond right or wrong. It forces you to explore the gray areas.

- Finally, challenge yourself to update your beliefs – and reward yourself when you do. It's the hallmark of a finely tuned mind.

So here's the real test. Did our little mind game work?

My guess is you still think carrots will improve your eyesight. That's okay. After all, I gave the same facts that are listed above to several folks over the last few days and, without exception, they all held on to their original belief.

Like I said, our brain plays powerful tricks on us.

But I urge you to spend time working to convince yourself of the truth. It will be much harder than you think. And if it's that hard to believe something different about something as diminutive as carrots, imagine how difficult the big issues will be.

But if you pull it off – if you manage to overcome one of mankind's greatest flaws – you'll be in better control of your thoughts and beliefs. You'll lead a much more fulfilled and successful life.

Plus, you'll know the truth about carrots.

A Life- and Health-Improving Mantra

J ohn Templeton is our kind of guy. The man made his money the honest way and used it to fund scientific research that will benefit us all.

You'll find what he learned about our brains equal parts fascinating and useful. But no essay on the man is complete without diving into his remarkable career as an investor.

We'll start there.

Templeton's story is one of timing. He borrowed some cash at the start of World War II and put it into the cheapest stocks he could find.

He bought a stake in 104 companies with share prices under a buck.

A full third of them were in bankruptcy.

It was a bold move... that we wouldn't recommend you mimic.

But, again, his timing was grand. All but four stocks paid off handsomely. He turned $10,000 into $40,000 in just four years.

Soon after counting his new pile of money, Templeton went into the mutual fund business, where he found great success.

He would eventually be knighted by Queen Elizabeth II and, perhaps just as noble, *Money* magazine argued he was the greatest stock picker of his time.

But the billionaire wasn't all about money.

He had a deep spiritual side that helped nourish his great philanthropic endeavors.

With the motto "How little we know, how eager to learn," our hero started the Templeton Foundation. Its mission was simply to grant money to folks eagerly studying new ideas.

In 1997, the effort spawned the Campaign for Forgiveness Research, a nonprofit aimed at taking a scientific – versus religious – approach to the idea of forgiveness.

What Templeton and his researchers found is a lesson for every man.

Forgiveness is one of the best medicines for our body and mind.

Forgive ~~and Forget~~

In experiment after experiment, the results were the same. When researchers asked participants to think about somebody they hold a grudge against – i.e., a person they have not forgiven – the folks doing the thinking underwent great physiological stress.

Their hearts beat faster. Their blood pressures surged. Their muscles tensed. And sweat dotted their brows.

No matter how long ago the unforgiven event happened, the body reacted quite negatively just to the thought of it.

Now imagine how many unforgiven things you carry with you right now.

Name them and feel your body fight back.

Failing to forgive puts tremendous stress on your body... stress that will shorten your life.

"When you don't forgive, you release all the chemicals of the stress response," says Stanford University's Dr. Frederic Luskin. "Each time you react, adrenaline, cortisol and norepinephrine enter the body. When it's a chronic grudge, you could think about it 20 times a day, and those chemicals limit creativity, they limit problem-solving. Cortisol and norepinephrine cause your brain to enter what we call 'the no-thinking zone,' and over time, they lead you to feel helpless and like a victim."

But there's a cure for this ailment.

In her book, *Triumph of the Heart: Forgiveness in an Unforgiving World*, author Megan Feldman Bettencourt reveals the research that proves all we must do is forgive, and the stress and the sludge of chemicals that come with it are gone.

So how do you do it? What's the trick?

After all, if forgiveness were so easy, religions wouldn't center on the idea and it wouldn't take dozens of multimillion-dollar research efforts to show us the dangerous nature of not letting go.

Step by Step

Thanks to a surge in research, brain docs have proven multiple ways to forgive others and release our minds from the shackles of angst.

Although they range from just one or two simple steps all the way to comprehensive 20-step programs, most proven forgiveness techniques contain the same basic four ideas.

First, we have to understand what we're holding on to.

What is it, and who is it that we have not forgiven?

In this foundational stage, we must reflect on failed attempts at forgiveness and why we failed.

From there, step two is making the conscious decision to forgive. It's not as easy as it sounds. It must be authentic, and we must be fully committed.

It's a step that trips a lot of wannabe forgivers.

Step three is quite emotional. It's where we confront the pain and work to understand it from other perspectives.

This is where, perhaps, we begin to see the other side of the story. It's where we contemplate the action from the perpetrator's point of view.

> The older we are, the easier it is to forgive and the more health benefits there are to forgiving.

Maybe the crook was trying to feed his starving family. Maybe he got hooked on drugs after hurting his back. Maybe he really is just a bad person.

Whatever the case, to fully forgive, we must fully understand. There are remarkable stories of forgiveness – and friendship – that have been bred from this critical process.

Finally, the last step is to simply reflect. It's where we examine the many ways the pain has affected our life. Many folks find solace in learning how similar instances affected others. Others simply ramble off a list of grievances.

No matter.

This is where we take whatever happened, admit that it changed our life, know that we're not the only one who's ever been wronged, crumple it all up and walk away.

We forgive.

Practice Helps

Finally, our age helps. Research shows that the older we are, the easier it is to forgive and the more health benefits there are to forgiving.

A study by Loren Toussaint of Iowa's Luther College proved a significant relationship between good health and forgiveness. But it was the folks over the age of 45 who appeared to gain the most. They reported far fewer feelings of sadness, anxiety and restlessness.

The concept is not hard to believe. Forgiveness takes practice.

But with age comes greater baggage. By failing to forgive, we harbor a lifetime of ill will. It builds up and affects our health.

Simply learn how to forgive, strive to do it every chance you get... and watch how your life and health improve.

Exercise Your Connections to Stay Healthy

The evidence is equal parts overwhelming and fascinating. There's a new chronic illness in America, and it's spreading like few scientists thought possible.

In fact, it's now thought that one of America's great forefathers suffered from the affliction... and our country took a different path because of it.

You see, when Thomas Jefferson returned home from his diplomatic duties in Europe, he had no plans to remain in the dirty world of politics. He went home to Monticello and planned to live out a peaceful, carefree retirement.

His plans were no different from the plans of most modern retirees.

But loneliness quickly set in. Jefferson had few callers and little interaction with the world outside of his vast estate.

It affected him greatly. His physical and mental health suffered quickly.

To overcome what ailed him, he knew he needed to return to Philadelphia and his vast network of social connections.

Once he did, his body and mind were quickly refreshed. Soon he was the vice president and then the president of a budding country.

It happened only because he got lonely... and he was smart enough to do something about it.

This idea is why "Connections" is the third leg of the Manward Triad. The folks we surround ourselves with and our interactions with them are key to leading rich, fulfilling lives.

Connect... or Face Serious Health Risks

Men often have a tough time admitting they're lonely, but very recent research shows just how deadly solitude can be.

If our Connections falter – the research shows – we may get to hang out with the Grim Reaper sooner than we'd like.

"Loneliness has surprisingly broad and profound health effects," said John T. Cacioppo, Ph.D., who was a professor at the University of Chicago and a leading voice on the topic. "Lonely people have more miserable lives and earlier deaths."

The health risks are off the charts. Loneliness has been linked to high blood pressure, sleep disorders, diabetes, Alzheimer's disease and dementia.

"There is robust evidence that social isolation and loneliness significantly increase risk for premature mortality, and the magnitude of the risk exceeds that of many leading health indicators," said Dr. Julianne Holt-Lunstad as she released new research at the 125th annual convention of the American Psychological Association.

She and her research team looked at more than 200 studies on the health effects of feeling alone and isolated.

Their conclusion stunned the medical world. Lonely people had a full 50% increased risk of death when compared with folks with strong social networks.

Compare that to the 30% rise in early death for obese folks. *Loneliness is now considered deadlier than obesity.* It's the equivalent, some sources say, of smoking 15 cigarettes a day.

"Being connected to others socially is widely considered a fundamental human need – crucial to both well-being and survival," the study concluded.

> Loneliness has been linked to high blood pressure, sleep disorders, diabetes, Alzheimer's disease and dementia.

What's crazy, though, is the rate that chronic loneliness seems to be storming through our society.

It's always been around, but it's turning out to be far more common in retiring baby boomers than in past generations.

One study showed that the number of folks who say they have no one to discuss important matters with rose from just 10% in 1985 to 24% in 2004... and to 35% today.

"The profound effects of loneliness on health and independence are a critical public health problem," said Dr. Carla M. Perissinotto, a geriatrician at the University of California. "It is no longer medically or ethically acceptable to ignore older adults who feel lonely and marginalized."

It's a major – and growing – problem in America.

"Social" Media Squashes Mental Health

We save for retirement. We eat healthy. We go to the gym.

But the vast majority of folks never bother to ponder the health of their social networks.

That's crazy.

In fact, for nearly half the nation's elderly population... TV is ranked as their main source of company.

We always said TV would kill you. Now we know why.

What's most concerning in all of this is that the notion of loneliness has become a cultural norm.

It's now quite easy and culturally acceptable to be on our own.

Marriage rates are on the decline. More couples than ever are deciding not to have children – a brave decision when they're young but potentially deadly as they age.

And hundreds of thousands of folks now go to work each day without ever leaving their living rooms or seeing another set of human eyes.

The consequences for our culture are not good.

Since the 1980s, for example, the average person's social network has shrunk by a third.

As technology advances, we need fewer folks in our lives. It leads to fewer friends... and fewer trusted Connections.

Lots of folks turn to social media to "connect" with their pals. But recent research even shows that idea is wrong.

Facebook admitted that social media can harm your mental health. Unless you're actively posting and messaging with your network, scrolling through social sites does far more harm than good. We need our Connections to stay healthy, successful and fulfilled.

A Major Breakthrough

We have one final piece of evidence to share with you: There's new data that shows loneliness is truly an affliction in our brains.

The fine folks at MIT recently published a study that shows an area of the brain long known as the home for depression is also a hot spot for chronic loneliness. It's called the dorsal raphe nucleus, and it does some crazy things.

In fact, when researchers studied loneliness in lab rats, they found that dopamine neurons in this section of the brain were inactive when the rats were housed together.

But when rats that had been isolated for just 24 hours were reintroduced with others, the neural activity surged.

It was a major breakthrough in the science of loneliness.

Science has clearly proven that being alone a lot is dangerous. Acute loneliness can kill.

To beat this affliction – and save your life – it's critical you **nurture your social relations**. Men especially need to be careful because our culture tends to put less weight on our need for an inner circle of companions.

The solution may seem obvious.

Exercise Your Connections

It starts, like so many of the ideas we explore at Manward, with education. Just knowing loneliness can kill is a key step. It should be the catalyst that pushes you forward.

From there, it's merely a matter of treating your Connections no differently than you would any form of exercise.

Make it a routine... and force yourself if necessary.

It doesn't matter how you do it. Some folks hang out at a coffee shop. Others spend time with family or get a part-time job.

But we also have a more nuanced fix... especially for men.

> Just as doctors urge us to get 150 minutes of exercise each week, be sure to get several hours' worth of social interaction each week.

Man-to-Man

You see, men don't respond as well as women to face-to-face interactions. Instead, we do better with shoulder-to-shoulder interactions.

It's why we volunteer hundreds of hours each year to be around like-minded men... doing like-minded activities.

It's why we can open the door to our woodshop, sit down with our old man, build something together with few words and walk away feeling much more connected (and healthier).

In Australia, men are flocking to a quickly growing social phenomenon called the Australian Men's Shed Association.

The concept is simple... get men together, working on stuff. It's attracted tens of thousands of men (it's gone international) who enhance their social networks by engaging in work that challenges their minds and their bodies. Little did these men know they were adding years to their lives.

Fight Back

If you're feeling lonely... if you feel like you're left out... if you've got nobody to talk to... or if you're using technology to feel connected...

we beg you to take action. Shoulder up with other men.

Your health will thank you. The Grim Reaper will move on to bug the next guy.

Yes, retirement is great. No more boss, no more daily grind and no more dealing with folks you may not be particularly fond of. But it's also a recipe for loneliness.

Thomas Jefferson realized it and fought back. It changed the course of American history.

What will you do when you get lonely?

Right This Wrong... That's Killing Us

T his is serious. Folks are dying. And 1 out of every 9 Americans is at risk.

We've looked into the connection between antidepressants and mass shootings in the past but never dove into it.

The waters were too rough.

But a man is blind if he doesn't know the facts.

So we'll dive right in, expand our Know-How and open our eyes.

The scene we see is a blurry mess.

Killer Dope

As with anything related to Big Pharma and therefore big money, the waters are muddy. Just as they start to clear up, somebody purposefully tosses in another bucket of dirt (at least we hope it's dirt).

Here's what we know right now.

The incidence of mass shootings in this country has risen right alongside the debut and booming popularity of antidepressants like Prozac.

Just about every headline-grabbing mass shooting was perpetrated by a mad white guy who was prescribed some sort of mind-altering drug.

There's no denying it.

But were these men (using the biological definition only) shooting up the world because they had serious mental issues (and were therefore taking drugs), or were they taking dangerous drugs that tricked them into making poor decisions?

The numbers are slowly moving in favor of the latter... which is scary. But there's a big problem if that's the case.

Get this... 1 in 9 Americans are now on some sort of antidepressant. We're home to the highest prescription rate on the planet.

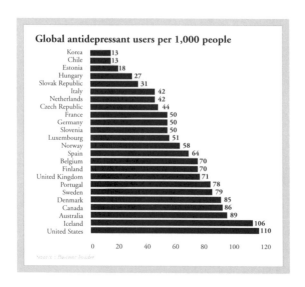

Some would argue that number alone explains why we're also home to the highest number of mass shootings... and wealthy drug salesmen.

But we beg caution.

Self-Help Leads to Self-Harm

Here's the thing. It's not the pills' tendency to drive a man to shoot up a theater that has us concerned.

It's their tendency to make us want to harm ourselves that must be studied and explained.

After all, isn't a mass shooting merely another atrocious form of suicide?

When it comes to that subject, the waters are far less muddy.

Many antidepressants come with an infamous "black box" warning that "children, adolescents and young adults" taking the drug have an increased risk of suicidal thinking and behavior.

We'll repeat... children, adolescents and young adults. The studies show that folks over age 24 are not at risk.

Do we need to remind readers the average age of the folks shooting up our schools and theaters?

But do we dare yank the pills off the shelves? Do we dare take our kids off drugs?

We can't.

The numbers are clear that suicide rates surge as soon as we get our kids off antidepressants.

In fact, shortly after the FDA made drugmakers put that infamous warning on their pills, antidepressant use among young people fell by 31%.

At the same time, suicide attempts by young adults surged by 34%.

In other words, our kids are in trouble no matter what.

Antidepressants, at least, save more lives than they take. The story here isn't all that much different than it is with guns.

The Answer

The conclusion is clear.

We must fulfill our **Triad**: Man up, get our hands dirty and figure out what's really going on here.

In other words, our nation must fix the problem that truly ails us... so we don't have to mask it with drugs.

That oh-so-slippery beast known as our culture is at play. We're focused on the wrong things.

If our culture weren't sick, we wouldn't need drugs.

If Hollywood didn't tout violence and sex...

If schools taught real life instead of politically correct propaganda...

And if men didn't flee the household...

We wouldn't need to wonder whether the drugs we use to fix the problem are killing us. We wouldn't need the drugs. It's our culture that's killing us. We say we are doing our share to right this wrong.

This little passion project of ours aims squarely at giving men the tools they need to stand firmly on their own two feet – without Big Pharma's toxins controlling their minds.

We know the answer to this problem (and think you do, too). We just need to convince the world.

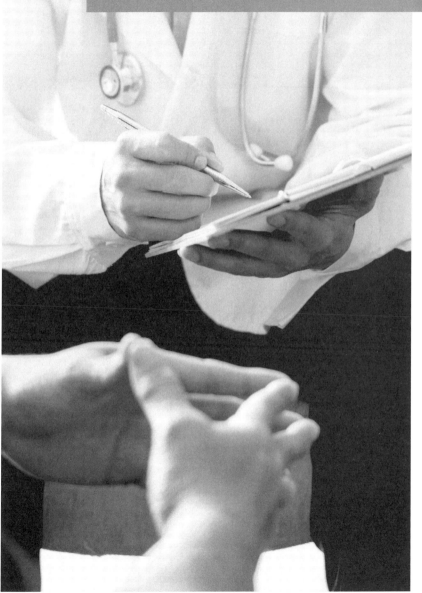

Down by 22%... The Danger Is All Around Us

I recently spent some time with my dad "off the grid." On the way home, I had a commitment at a shooting range that would take several hours.

I tossed the keys to my truck to my father and told him to pick me up in four hours.

I shot a hundred rounds or so, qualified to carry a badge and a gun for another year, and met my ride at the gate just after sunset.

"Where in the world did you go?" I asked as I looked at the fuel gauge.

"I drove down to the college to get some ice cream," he replied, knowing I'd be jealous of the big-name school's famed creamery.

"How was it?"

"Great," he said. "But, jeez, college kids are not what they used to be...

"The men," he said, putting air quotes around the last word, "are so geeky."

Bam... he said what we've all been thinking.

But what's crazy is that he's right.

Science has given us overwhelming evidence that today's men are, well, less manly than men of yesteryear.

What's worse is that your manliness meter may be falling too.

The crazy phenomenon has serious health consequences – even for women.

A Stunning Drop

Studies have shown that modern fruits and vegetables contain less vitamins and nutrients than they did just 50 years ago.

In some cases, the difference is stunning.

They're a fraction of what they used to be. It's not good.

What's worse, though, is the same sort of decline is happening to us humans.

Get this.

A study of men in the U.S. showed a shocking 22% drop in testosterone levels in the few decades between 1987 and 2004.

That's scary. And it's not some statistical anomaly.

The study was simple and accurate. Starting in 1987, researchers selected random men, between the ages of 45 and 79, living in and around Boston.

Those men set the baseline. The researchers then performed two follow-up studies of men of the same age from the same location. Those tests ended in 1997 and 2004.

The results were not good.

Again, by 2004, testosterone had dropped by 22%. The researchers concluded with this:

> We observe a substantial age-independent decline in [testosterone] that does not appear to be attributable to observed changes in explanatory factors, including health and lifestyle characteristics such as smoking and obesity.

A doctor from the New England Research Institutes put it in simpler terms:

> In 1988, men who were 50 years old had higher serum testosterone concentrations than did comparable 50-year-old men in 1996. This suggests that some factor other than age may be contributing to the observed declines in testosterone over time.

In other words, they know what's happening... and the reasons why are scary.

Chemical Soup

There's growing evidence that much of America's drinking water is polluted.

It's laced with traces of industrial and pharmaceutical chemicals that are slowly attacking our bodies.

And it's not just our testosterone levels that are out of whack.

For the last 40 years, scientists have quietly worried about declining sperm counts. Study after study showed trouble was brewing.

But it's research released just last year that shows the truly awful conclusion.

This study detailed the findings of 138 reports submitted between 1980 and 2015.

This granddaddy of all research projects sorted the good from the bad... it tossed tainted results... and it accounted for regional variations.

The results are startling.

Sperm counts in men across the globe plunged by 57% during the 35-year test period.

Clearly, we're losing the war against our manhood. (Women should pay attention too.)

Man... That Hurts

This is critical research because testosterone is linked to our health in so many ways.

Just a bit of Know-How on the subject could, at best, save our lives.

At worst, it could greatly enhance our everyday health.

In the simplest terms, testosterone is the hormone of virility.

It's what makes a man... a man. It puts hair on our chests. It builds our muscles.

And it boosts the size of our, well... suffice it to say, it's what makes a man a man.

But women depend on the chemical too. It's just as important that they keep their "T" levels in check.

It's the hormone behind more than 200 functions in women – like maintaining bone health and managing pain.

What's important to understand – no matter your sex – is that by the time we turn 30, our testosterone levels are on the decline.

It's a natural process. But there are things we can do about it.

The symptoms of low "T" are clear. We've known them for a while:

- Fatigue
- Low sex drive
- Increased body fat
- Decreased body hair
- Loss of strength and/or muscle mass
- Sleeping problems
- Depression.

But when it comes to knowing what causes low "T," scientists are just now learning that environmental factors are at work.

It turns out where we live is often an important factor in our testosterone levels.

Get this. In one of the scariest examples, researchers studied a group of Native Americans living on land that neighbors a large chemical plant.

For years, the Chippewas of Aamjiwnaang had normal birth levels.

The percentage of male births on the reservation from 1989 to 1993 was 55.1% – perfectly normal.

But when researchers came back a decade later, the level had fallen to just 34.8%.

Scientists blamed the chemical factory and its effect on hormones in the womb.

What's happened to the Chippewas is one of the most drastic examples of the environmental epidemic.

But the same decline in male birth rates is evident amongst a much larger sample population.

In fact, compared with 1970, there are 21 fewer males per 10,000 births. It's a small decline, but it's statistically relevant... and it's cause for concern. Big concern.

Again, doctors are looking at our environment and the food we eat.

Don't Drink That

The problem is there are dangerous chemicals and drugs all around us.

For example, in one recent study, 90% of men had evidence of chlorpyrifos in their urine.

Because the powerful ingredient in pesticides and fertilizers is poured onto nearly everything we eat, our diet is the main source of the chemical.

What's alarming is the men with the highest levels had about 20% less testosterone than those with lower exposure.

That's scary. Most folks have no idea what's happening.

But it gets worse.

I spend hundreds of volunteer hours each year working on conservation efforts. One of those efforts focuses on one of the East Coast's largest – and sickest – rivers.

The Susquehanna River flows through some nasty areas. In its headwaters, acid runoff from long gone coal mining operations infects the water. Many of the river's feeder streams still aren't fit for life.

Downstream, the mighty river flows by town after town... each adding a bit more pollution.

By the time the river finally dumps into the Chesapeake Bay, its water contains a whole lot more than hydrogen and oxygen.

One area of particular concern is sewer effluence. It's a leading suspect in the hormone morass.

You see, modern sewage plants are quite good at cleaning natural waste from our sewers.

But they simply can't eradicate the artificial chemicals that we push into – and therefore out of – our bodies.

It's the reason – at least according to a growing group of scientists – that fish in the Susquehanna River are growing organs of both sexes.

That's right... hermaphroditic bass. Experts blame a wide array of synthetic drugs... including birth control pills.

Sewage plants simply can't eradicate the synthetic hormones in the pills. With one popular birth control compound, scientists found that up to 68% of each dose eventually goes down the toilet.

And researchers at Harvard tell us that just a single dose of testosterone cream can put as much of the hormone into the water as the natural excretion of 300 men.

So with each flush, estrogen- and testosterone-manipulating drugs build up in our waterways.

What's even worse is flushing unused drugs down the toilet.

It's another major problem that, interestingly, makes nursing homes a rather unknown, yet dangerous, source of pollution. They're notorious for flushing unused prescriptions.

Of course, the folks making the drugs are a problem too.

While studying why male fish are suddenly turning into females, the U.S. Geological Survey found pollution levels 10 to 1,000 times higher than average downstream of pharmaceutical plants.

Go figure.

And let's not forget the hormones we're sticking into our dinner in the name of creating a nicely marbled steak.

Farms are quickly being recognized as major sources of hormonal pollution.

It makes sense.

Farmers inject their animals with growth hormones, much of which goes straight into the waste stream. From there, it ends up on a field and washes into drinking water.

It all adds up to big trouble. Our water is poisonous.

You've likely never heard of the study, but the Associated Press published test results of water samples from 24 major cities that, you guessed it, showed detectable levels of pharmaceuticals in them.

A similar study of 19 treatment plants found antidepressants, antipsychotics, antibiotics, beta-blockers and tranquilizers.

It's no wonder one generation after the next is becoming – getting right to our point – less and less manly.

Our environment is toxic... and it threatens the very nature of man.

The scientific community is quickly realizing we face a big problem, especially when it comes to falling levels of testosterone.

The Natural Solution

Fortunately, there's plenty that we can do to fight the problem... without asking our doctor for a prescription.

It starts with our diet.

Modern man's diet is simply a disaster. It's processed. It's packed with drugs. And the nutrients have been virtually bred out in the name of faster, more efficient growth.

Our research shows that a diet that's optimized for testosterone production must focus on minimizing carbohydrates. The data is interesting. It shows that a diet high in carbs – the typical American diet – leads to elevated levels of insulin secretion.

> Two effective, natural ways to boost testosterone levels are to eat more vegetables and to exercise.

All that insulin lowers "T" production.

What's crazy is that it takes nearly a full year on a **low-carb diet** to bring insulin levels back to where they belong.

A quicker way to boost your body's natural production is to eat more **vegetables**, especially those with high levels of vitamin D and zinc.

A recent study showed that taking 3,300 international units of **vitamin D** each day increased testosterone levels.

The correlation between the vitamin and the hormone was clear... one leads to the other.

The same research shows that foods with high levels of **D-aspartic acid** – like **almonds**, **eggs** and **lentils** – are also good "T" boosters.

And here's one that hurts... beer has been shown to hurt "T" levels. In fact, in one study, the estrogenlike properties of hops were shown to lower testosterone by nearly 7%.

That's enough that some doctors are now exploring using hops to help women with menopause-induced hot flashes.

Crazy.

Finally, it's no surprise that **exercise** is one of the most effective ways to boost hormone levels.

One six-second fix is to simply **sprint**. The *International Journal of Sports Medicine* found that a quick sprint significantly boosted "T" levels – even long after the exercise was over.

It's a similar situation with lifting. **Resistance training** stimulates strong levels of testosterone production.

The trick with using exercise to boost levels of the key hormone is to understand that it takes short, intense exercise... not prolonged aerobic exercise.

The ideal "T"-boosting exercise would look like this:

- Warm up for three to five minutes.
- Exercise as hard and fast as possible for 30 seconds (go all out).
- Recover for 60 to 90 seconds.
- Repeat the exercise and recovery process seven more times.
- Cool down for three to five minutes.

The whole process takes less than half an hour. And not only has it been proven to boost testosterone levels, but it also gives us a heart-healthy exercise that will boost our mental well-being.

Do it at least three times each week.

Fighting for Mankind

Modern life is not treating men well. We're sedentary. Our diet is poisonous. And our environment is riddled with dangerous chemicals.

It's nearly impossible to escape all that threatens us.

From the water we drink to the plastics that envelop nearly everything we consume... testosterone is surrounded by its mortal enemies.

It's affecting us. It's affecting mankind.

The evidence is overwhelming. Fish are growing two sets of sex organs. Male birth rates are falling. And, like my father said, today's men just aren't what they used to be.

It's an epidemic we must fight. And it's a fight we must win.

The Toxic Reason Prostate Cancer Is Soaring

M en are under attack. It's a slow assault that's gone virtually un-noticed. But we're surrounded.

Our environment is toxic... It's killing the very idea of manhood.

We're surrounded by chemicals. They're in the food we eat... they're in our cars... they're in our bedrooms... they're even leeching out of cash register receipts.

They're called **xenoestrogens** – or, using our knowledge of Greek roots, "foreign" estrogen.

Simply put, these chemicals mimic estrogen.

When they find their way into our bodies, they trigger the same sort of response that natural estrogen would.

Obviously, that can cause some problems... especially for men.

The effect on our prostate is a prime example.

This critical "manly" organ reacts to the estrogen our bodies normally produce.

Once the receptors are triggered, the prostate is signaled to do what it does.

But when xenoestrogen gets to the prostate, the same signals are fired.

Put simply, it confuses our bodies.

It can lead to an overgrown prostate, inflammation and, a subject too many men are quickly learning about these days, prostate cancer.

> *Xenoestrogens ("foreign" estrogens)*: Natural or synthetic hormones that mimic estrogen and disrupt the body's endocrine system, causing a wide range of health problems.

Research released last year showed that metastatic prostate cancer climbed 72% in the decade prior to 2013. For men between the critical ages of 55 and 69... instances of the deadly disease rose 92%.

There's no doubt xenoestrogens played a leading role in this surge of cancer.

You Gonna Eat That?

Avoiding the onslaught of nasty chemicals is nearly impossible. Like we said, they're all around us... and in our water.

But there are a few key things you can do to minimize your exposure.

First, treat plastic like the enemy. It's most folks' No. 1 source of xenoestrogen.

You'll likely recall the big BPA scare several years ago. The food industry was shaken when it was told to get the nasty cancer-causing chemical out of its products.

But guess what... BPA is still around. And so are several other just-as-nasty chemicals.

The worst thing we can do is heat our food in plastic. Some containers can take the heat... many cannot.

Those that can't put off some horrific chemicals when put in the microwave or, yes, the dishwasher.

Get this... Xenoestrogen-containing plastics leech chemicals in your dishwasher – coating every other dish in the load.

Again, avoid eating anything from a plastic container.

Another chemical to watch for is propyl gallate, a preservative that's been in our food for nearly 70 years. Look for it in the ingredient list of your favorite factory-fresh foods.

It's in our candy... our processed meats and potatoes... and our snack foods.

Avoid it... research proves it does weird (and possibly deadly) things to our bodies.

As always, the best way to win this war is to eat as naturally as possible. Avoid processed foods. Stay away from factory-farmed meat. And absolutely don't eat out of heated plastic.

Your manhood depends on it.

Face Your Fears and Get Informed

For men, prostate cancer is something to fear. For Big Pharma, it's something to cheer.

With nearly 200,000 fresh cases diagnosed each year, prostate cancer is the fourth most common form of cancer.

With such big numbers, it's no surprise when our sources reveal just how fierce the battle for market share has become.

There's big money on the line... very big money.

Fighting prostate cancer is quickly becoming one of the most lucrative games in the healthcare business.

Big Pharma = Big Prostate

The numbers speak for themselves.

In 2016, for example, the treatment market was valued at just over $5.6 billion. But recent research shows that, by 2025, sales will surge past $18 billion annually.

So in less than nine years...

The market will have more than tripled.

Few other industries are working in such lush pastures.

With so much money on the line, companies jumping into the battle against prostate cancer have been rewarded handsomely.

They fight hard to keep every inch of ground they've won.

A prime example came from Johnson & Johnson in early 2018...

The FDA approved the company's latest prostate cancer fighter, called Erleada. Designed to bust up tumors that aren't responding to traditional treatments, it's the first drug of its kind to get the nod from the nation's healthcare regulator.

As any investor in the space will tell you, an FDA win is rare... and expensive.

But Johnson & Johnson knows patients – and their insurers – are willing to pay.

A single 120-tablet bottle of the newly approved drug comes with a $10,920 price tag.

Fighting cancer is big money.

That's why the news of the win with the FDA came at the perfect time.

No-Name Competition

Just as Erleada was making a big – and lucrative – move forward, Johnson & Johnson was losing patent coverage on its blockbuster prostate cancer drug.

A U.S. court tossed out the patent that keeps Zytiga free from competition. It opens the field to generic makers of the drug and their cheap pills.

It will hurt.

Zytiga raked in $2.5 billion in sales for Johnson & Johnson in 2017 alone.

Unless the high-priced lawyers at the company sway the judge at their upcoming appeal, much of that money could soon be going to generic competitors.

What's scary in all of this is that despite treatment breakthroughs, the instances of deadly metastatic prostate cancer continue to climb.

In the decade between 2004 and 2013, for instance, the number of new cases soared by more than 70%.

And the odds of a man getting prostate cancer are now higher than ever.

It makes us scratch our head and ponder something.

We wonder – with so many billions of dollars on the line – are the big drug companies secretly rejoicing? Are they happy to see their market expanding by the day?

Clearly prostate cancer is something to fear.

But for drug companies, it's something to cheer.

It's vital that men understand all sides of this common form of cancer.

It's Know-How that could save your life... and your wallet.

The Simple Decision That Is Killing Men

The grave and growing risk from prostate cancer is proof that Big Government should stick to doing what it does best... gerrymandering, bickering and reaching into our pockets.

Folks who have paid attention aren't surprised by the latest data.

They predicted this would happen half a decade ago.

They foresaw one simple decision costing the lives of countless men.

Our story begins where so many stories of its kind begin. We can only imagine some vote-hungry politician getting a call from an angry constituent.

He hangs up the phone and quickly demands a panel... perhaps even a blue-ribbon panel.

The voter is happy... he got heard.

The swamp dweller is happy... he'll get a vote.

And the panel participants are happy... they got a fresh fistful of taxpayer dollars.

Death Panels

This was the scene in 2012 when the U.S. Preventive Services Task Force got together to discuss the oh-so-squirmy topic of prostate cancer testing.

They took aim at the most popular detection tool, known as the prostate specific antigen (PSA) test. After talking it through – at least we hope they talked – the group said the test did more harm than good.

Insurance providers rejoiced.

Funeral homes toasted the news.

Business was going up.

The task force looked at reams of data and determined that the side effects of the PSA – impotency, incontinence, unnecessary radiation and added costs (don't forget the costs…) – outweighed the benefit of the test.

For every life saved, the Big Government-funded panel decreed, dozens more were harmed…

It led to headlines like this one from *The Washington Post*: "Government task force discourages routine testing for prostate cancer."

Cancer fighters across the country cried foul. Surely, they claimed, this would lead to a rise in men dying of cancer.

That was five years ago… five years before we got a headline like this one: "Prostate Cancer Deaths on the Rise."

And this one: "New Government PSA Testing Guidelines Are Flawed and Dangerous for Men's Health."

And this one: "Men Are Dying Too Young From Prostate Cancer."

Most of the articles point to a fact that many doctors tried to raise five years ago.

They predicted that with less screening, more men would end up dying of cancer because they'd find it too late.

After all, prostate cancer has few symptoms.

Their predictions rang true in a study released in 2016 in the journal *Prostate Cancer and Prostatic Diseases.*

It reveals that the rates of metastatic prostate cancer – the nasty kind that spreads and kills – have risen 72% in the last 10 years. Worse, the rate surged to 92% for men between 55 and 69 years old.

"These recent trends highlight the continued need for nationwide refinement in prostate cancer screening and treatment to prevent the morbidity and mortality associated with metastatic prostate cancer," the researchers wrote in the study.

"The burden of overtreatment and side effects may no longer be sufficient to recommend against routine screening," said Dr. Jim Hu, the Cornell professor who recently completed another study on the subject.

"The public health message is that after years of decline, the incidence of metastatic disease has gone up," he added. "And while the PSA test is not perfect, I don't think people should be told that this test has no value."

Sorry 'Bout Dat

After viewing these life-destroying figures, Uncle Sam's blue-ribbon panel convened once again.

The "experts" put their heads together, deliberated on the best way to get themselves out of the jam and made a new decree.

It turns out **PSA screenings** have a "small advantage for some men."

The panel now advises doctors to "offer or provide this service for selected patients depending on individual circumstances."

We're not sure what the panel meant by "individual circumstances," but we imagine it may have to do with the patient's ability to sue... or at least his connections to a few good lawyers.

Our point here isn't to give medical advice. Our medical Know-How ends at how to skin a rabbit.

Instead we beg readers to go into the exam room with a wary eye.

The press won't cover it (it'd be akin to admitting their handlers in Washington were wrong), but 27,000 men will die from prostate cancer this year. And thanks, at least in part, to reduced screening, that number will be up significantly from last year's.

That's why we do our homework. It's why we value an array of opinions. And it's why we don't trust anybody with our life – especially if their lifestyle depends on our vote.

This is serious stuff.

Get informed and spread the word.

It may just save a life.

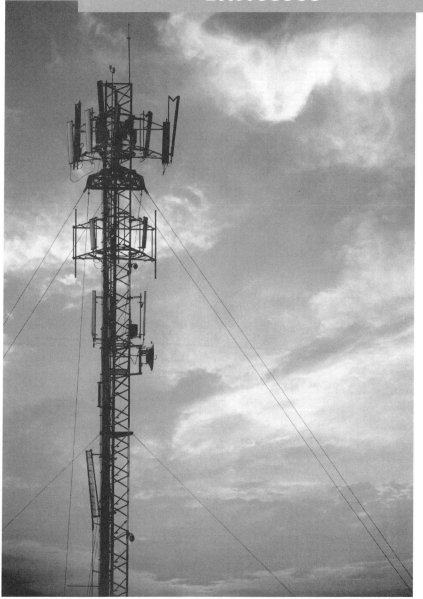

Part VI: 21st-Century Illnesses

How Modern Technology Creates Serious Health Problems

D o you suffer from unexplained headaches, fatigue, depression or skin irritation?

Have you or a loved one recently been diagnosed with an autoimmune disease? If so, there may be a new culprit in your home. Or, worse, it may be leaking from your neighbor's home.

It's the result of technology moving faster than our healthcare system.

What's most surprising, though, is that the culprit may just be the things that so many folks think are doing so much good.

Before we go there, though, we need to cover the basics.

No Standards

As capacitors started to find their way into more and more of the nation's electrical equipment in the 1970s, electronics manufacturers and power providers quickly realized they needed some sort of standard.

Without it, the various frequencies of electricity shooting through our power lines could wreak havoc on sensitive equipment.

The result was something known as IEEE 519. It's an industry code that ensures the electricity that flows into our houses is clean and standardized.

If you plug in a computer in Burbank, the electrical charge (the frequency, the voltage, etc.) is the same as it is in Bismarck.

The code – even though it never became law – works quite well.

The juice flowing into our houses is very clean.

But, thanks to all sorts of new (i.e., untested) technology in our homes, we're seeing a much different trend as the electricity flows throughout our home and its equipment. For some folks, it's causing serious health problems.

Silent Killer

Jeromy Johnson is one of them.

"My wife and I," he recently explained on a podcast, "we had a bank of smart meters, the wireless smart meters that measure electricity, put right below our bedroom in San Francisco. Within a week, we couldn't sleep, had headaches, heart palpitations and ringing in the ears."

Again, he blames the rapid – untested – onslaught of fresh technology.

"The old ones that we've had for almost a hundred years, they had a dial on them," Johnson said. "The company would come out and write down your measurements once a month. The new ones communicate wirelessly, and they send that data back to the company. Sounds like a good idea. I'm an environmentalist. I did think that this could be a good idea, but what they've done is they've made those meters so they send sometimes 10,000, up to almost 200,000 pulses of microwave radiation each day."

What's crazy is that Johnson said he now can't be near a cell tower for very long. He doesn't use Wi-Fi. And he refuses to own a smartphone.

Doctors admit the symptoms of this "electromagnetic allergy" are real. It's a real syndrome.

In fact, in a landmark case, France is paying a 39-year-old woman roughly $900 a month in disability payments because of her fight with the ailment.

But docs continue to say there isn't enough evidence to draw any real scientific conclusions.

The symptoms, they say, are too universal.

How do we know if a headache is caused by stress or an errant Wi-Fi router? How do we know a cellphone caused that man's testicular cancer?

> **Electromagnetic allergy:** A sensitivity to electromagnetic field sources that can cause unexplained headaches, dizziness, skin irritation and fatigue.

It's still too early in the game for docs to raise a red flag... not enough folks are connecting the dots between their symptoms and what's causing them.

But that hasn't stopped researchers like Johnson (who's written a book on the subject) and Alison Main from pushing the idea to the masses.

Main recently wrote an article for a major health publication. In it, she took a detailed look at the newfangled products in our homes that are operating outside the accepted IEEE 519 code.

She points to things like CFL bulbs, LED lighting, wireless routers and even solar energy systems... anything that distorts electrical harmonics.

"The problem with most energy-efficient appliances and light bulbs," she writes, "are the switch-mode power supplies that are used to reduce voltage and convert from AC to DC. This process distorts the otherwise-smooth sine wave of 60 hertz AC, producing harmonics that then radiate along your wires and penetrate your living space."

Of course, electronics manufacturers aren't going to change their ways if doctors aren't yet willing to put their stamp on the problem.

That means it's up to consumers to become knowledgeable about the problem and, most important, to do something about it.

The solution is simple.

Unplug.

Avoid devices that provide this sort of harmonic distortion. Use Wi-Fi sparingly. Turn it off while you sleep. Keep your bed away from charging devices. And limit the amount of time you're on your phone.

Just as important, if you are experiencing the symptoms above, take good notes. Write down when you feel sick and keep track of what sorts of devices or appliances are close by when the symptoms are at their worst.

Some folks have likened today's problem to the air pollution boom of the 1970s and '80s. We built smokestack after smokestack as we rushed to take advantage of the nation's industrial might.

But as the rush slowed, we realized there was a downside... a very unhealthy, cancer-causing downside.

We say the problem we face today also has eerie parallels to the cancer cover-up perpetrated by Big Tobacco a generation ago. The problem was clear... but the money was good.

Folks died while others got rich. Eventually, though, the truth came out. Will we someday regret the convenience of Wi-Fi, smartphones and a world where everything is connected?

Perhaps some folks will... but not us. We're taking action now – before we get sick.

The Deadly Truth About This Cover-Up

Have we been lied to? Have we been misled by an industry that's more concerned with profits than the health of its customers?

It surely wouldn't be the first time.

The tobacco industry pulled the wool over the world's eyes for more than a decade before the whispers got too loud to quiet. And the fine folks at Facebook have been taking heat for covering up quite the long-running scandal.

But we're tracking something even bigger... a cover-up that runs deep within an industry that's worth, get this, *half a trillion dollars* annually.

It's no wonder the folks on the inside are trying to kick dust over the growing stream of bad news.

But the whispers are starting to turn into shouts... shouts that we're convinced the rest of the world will soon hear.

Cancer Scare

We first told of the nasty link between cellphones and cancer in 2017.

Since then, a growing community of doctors and researchers have been waving their arms, warning consumers to pay attention. Their studies prove something is amiss.

But there is a problem.

Most of the studies until recently were paid for by the cellphone industry.

And, imagine this, the instant any sort of bad news erupted, the studies were pulled and the researchers were fired.

It made it tough to explore the truth.

"Everyone knows that if your research results show that radiation has effects, the funding flow dries up," said Dariusz Leszczynski, a biochemistry researcher at the University of Helsinki, in 2011.

He shouldn't have said anything.

A year later, his own study was pulled and he was out of a job.

But there's a fresh study these days that's outside the reach of "Big Wireless"...

Here's what we've written about it:

> *This new research from the National Institutes of Health (NIH) is downright scary.*
>
> *A two-year, $25 million study showed that when rats were blasted with radiofrequency radiation (just like our phones produce), their chances of cancer soared off the charts.*
>
> *But here's the craziest part of the new study... the effect was seen only in male rats.*

At that point, the NIH had released only partial results. Why hit us with all the bad news at once, right?

It promised a full report later.

Well... we got it.

Ruh-Roh

The top cellular radiation researchers from across the planet flew to North Carolina recently to discuss the latest findings.

The result?

"Surprising" was the word we saw used most often. There was stunningly clear evidence connecting phone radiation and tumors in the rats tested in the study.

In fact, a panel of leading researchers voted that the results of the testing were "more significant than originally thought."

"The heart tumors are of a type that have been shown to be elevated in some epidemiology studies of humans who have used their cellphones under the highest power conditions for the longest period of time," said John Bucher of the National Institute of Environmental Health Sciences.

> A recent study shows there's stunningly clear evidence connecting phone radiation and tumors.

What this new research and the scientific community's backing of it means for the shady cellphone industry, we don't know.

But we know it will be big... and expensive.

There are "many brain tumor lawsuits going on right now that are waiting for a study like this to prove that people's brain tumors were caused by their cellphone radiation," said Kevin Mottus of the California Brain Tumor Association.

The FDA has now promised to take a look at the data.

Getting Worse

Meanwhile, the nation and its cancer docs are getting ready for a brand-new and far more powerful cellular technology to hit the airwaves this year.

The new 5G system promises to be stronger than anything that's currently available. But because of the nature of its short-lived signal, it will require more transmitters than the current network.

In other words, if cellphones are causing cancer in humans... we haven't seen anything yet.

As we double down on the amount of radiation in the air and the power behind it, our health is at greater risk than ever.

Do we think the big cellphone companies are going to tell us about it?

No way.

At least, not until well after folks start dropping over dead.

If Zuckerberg couldn't admit to a security breach until long after it happened... there's no way his pals at Apple and the like are going to step in front of this speeding train.

We've been lied to. We've been misled.

But the truth is slowly coming out... one new tumor at a time.

17 Simple, Lifesaving Tricks to Break a Killer Habit

A re the electronic products in your home killing you? If you've been paying attention, you know the answer is yes.

If you spent one-third of your day exposed to secondhand smoke that could give you lung cancer... you'd certainly do something about it.

If you spent a third of your day exposed to an infectious disease... you'd take action to avoid infection. But when it comes to our beloved electronic devices... we ignore the facts.

The average person spends *one-third of their day* glued to a cellphone, laptop or tablet. *And as we've mentioned, your cellphone, in particular – regardless of which company made it – is emitting dangerous levels of radiation.*

The facts are alarming...

More than 15,000 studies show that radiation emitted from phones has an adverse effect on human tissue.

And the World Health Organization has declared that cellphones damage your memory, your hearing, your skin and, yes, even your genitals.

Studies show it, doctors recognize it, and even the phone manufacturers acknowledge it.

It turns out – due to the levels of dangerous radiation coming out of your phone – Apple and other manufacturers *must legally tell you* to never hold the phone to your body when in use. And they have... sort of. They've buried the warnings deep in obscure sections of the owner's manuals. In Apple's case, I found it on Page 184.

When you talk on your cellphone (or use your computer), you're zapping your body with radiofrequency (RF) radiation.

There are dozens of studies, facts and examples showing that RF radiation warps living tissue, damages DNA, and promotes tumor growth and diseases like cancer.

But here's the thing... nobody knows what 20 to 30 years of close-proximity radiation exposure are going to do to us, as most of these products have been widely used for only 10 to 15 years.

However, based on what we've discovered... it's not a pretty picture.

Your cellphone and other electronic devices are very likely causing you harm in one way or another. But that harm can be prevented.

Here's how.

Use a Radiation Redirector

My No. 1 way to beat harmful radiation is to use a **radiation redirector** that attaches directly to your cellphone case.

This product redirects radiation energy from the face of the cellphone toward the back of the device. This significantly reduces the amount of radiation that would typically travel directly toward your head.

The technology used was originally developed to protect fetuses in the womb. It's the result of 10 years of research and experimentation in the science of electromagnetic wave modulation.

That might sound complicated, but the beauty of a product like this lies in its simplicity; stick it on... and forget it.

When you attach a redirector to your cellphone case, <u>less than one-tenth (in some cases, less than one-thirty-fifth) of the radiation's original strength reaches your head</u>. This tool is also able to redirect the radiation without any loss of signal strength.

There is credible evidence to show that this device does what it's intended to do: keep radiation away from your body.

So if you absolutely must talk on your cellphone (or wear it on your body), use a radiation-protective device.

That way, when you are talking on the phone with it held up against your ear, the device is redirecting radiation away from your head and body, where it could otherwise cause serious damage.

One product I recommend is the WaveSafe, which is available on Amazon. But do your own due diligence, and pay attention to what you are purchasing.

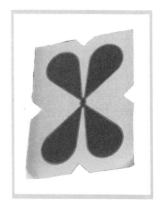

New research shows that some standard cellphone cases can actually increase radiation exposure by up to 70%.

Fortunately, there are cases that have been designed to protect against radiation, like SilverShield, DefenderShield and Pong.

Look for a product's SAR (specific absorption rate) value. You want a shielding device that blocks the most radiation.

(SAR is a measure of the rate at which energy is absorbed by a body exposed to radiation.)

A radiation redirector is a huge step toward a healthier future for you and your family.

But that's just the first step – laptops, tablets and cordless phones are also giving off harmful radiation. The average American home now has an average of seven active connected devices in use every day, potentially filling your body with deadly waves of radiation.

That's why I want to give you as many ways as possible to protect yourself.

And it's why I'm including an additional 11 ways to fight killer radiation.

This list includes some of the very basic, easy things you can do to lower your exposure. These are all things you should be doing... but likely are not.

Turn Your Phone Off More Often and/or Limit Its Electrical Output

First of all, when the device is off, no radiation is emitted. So, obviously, that is the safest thing you can do.

But since that is not always practical, you can reduce the radiation output with this simple fix: Your phone's screen is where a lot of the radiation is coming from, so turn it down.

On the iPhone, drag your finger upward from the bottom of the screen to make the Control Center appear. The box with a sun image controls the screen brightness. On an Android phone, open Settings, and tap Display, then Brightness. Turn off Automatic Brightness, then use the slider to dim the brightness manually.

Consider Alternative Methods of Communication

When possible, **send text messages** instead of making or receiving a call for which you put the phone against your head. The farther you can keep the phone from your body... the better. Anything is better than pressing it against your head. Also consider using a landline or Skype, which offers ways to stay in touch without a cellphone.

Switch to Airplane Mode Even on the Ground

Switch the phone to **airplane mode** when you give your cellphone to your kids to play with, especially toddlers. In airplane mode, the phone is using a lot less energy and emitting a lot less radiation. When there's no cell signal, the phone pours even more power into its antenna, trying to find a signal.

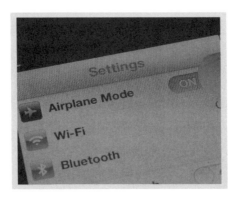

This creates even more radiation. So instead of putting your phone in your pocket and blasting yourself with radiation – put your phone on airplane mode.

On the iPhone, swipe your finger up from the bottom of the screen to open the Control Center. Tap the top left icon, which will be a picture of an airplane. On Android, open Settings; then, under Connections, tap Airplane Mode.

Protect Yourself and Sleep Well

One common practice is using a cellphone as an alarm clock and keeping it on the bedside table. Unfortunately, this places the phone near the head, where the radiation will do the most damage.

At night, put your phone on airplane mode or keep it on the other side of the bedroom. Although airplane mode disconnects the phone from Wi-Fi, the phone is still emitting low levels of radiation from the battery.

Turning off your phone or leaving it in another room is an even better solution. Even when off, your phone is still collecting phone calls and text messages. They'll all be there when you wake up in the morning and turn your phone back on.

Plus, you'll get a good night's sleep without waking up to the pinging sound of incoming messages.

Opt for the Convenience and Safety of Speakerphone

I've discussed the many health issues that close proximity to your cellphone creates.

Cellphone usage is being directly linked to the outbreak of cancer of the parotid gland. Holding a cellphone to your ear exposes your salivary glands to radiation.

Research has shown a fourfold increase in cancer of the parotid gland over a recent 35-year period. While rates of other salivary gland cancers stayed the same, cancer of the parotid gland – which is located closest to your cheek – skyrocketed.

Using speakerphone significantly reduces the radiation that penetrates your brain.

Get Plugged In

You want to keep your vital organs – particularly your face and brain – as far away from your phone as possible. When you hold the phone to your ear, the radiation is concentrated near your brain. **Using a headset** when speaking on the phone significantly reduces the radiation that penetrates your brain.

Also, because radiation may still travel through the wire, buy a ferrite bead to attach to the wire. The bead absorbs radiation traveling through the wire.

Again, for obvious reasons, **texting** is greatly preferable to calling when it comes to minimizing the concentration of radiation around the vulnerable brain.

Turn Off Background Updating and "Push" Data

Some cellphone apps frequently check the internet for new information – Facebook, Twitter, stock-reporting apps and so on – producing additional radiation and causing harm to your body.

You can turn off the background updating feature for individual apps. On the iPhone, tap Settings, then General, then Background App Refresh. You'll see an on/off switch for each app.

There's no similar feature on Android. But some Android phones offer features called Extreme Power Saver or Ultra Power Saver, which turn off background app updating.

"Push" email, which makes new messages appear in real time, is another serious radiation generator. What's happening, of course, is that your phone is checking for messages *every second*, which uses power.

The more power that is used, the more radiation emitted. On the iPhone, you can tap Settings, then Passwords & Accounts, then Fetch

New Data, then turn off Push. On Android, you may need to adjust this setting individually for each app.

Be Aware of Your "Bars"

Your phone uses radio waves to connect to Wi-Fi hotspots and wireless Bluetooth gadgets. It's constantly searching for the best connections. The harder it works to make those connections, the more radiation it emits.

Cellphones with better reception transmit at lower power than those that need to work harder. Whenever possible, use your cellphone only when you have full connectivity bars. These indicate a good, strong signal.

Or try to **go without Wi-Fi and Bluetooth** features when possible. On the iPhone, you'll find the on/off switches in the Control Center. On an Android phone, tap Settings; the on/off switches are right at the top. (As an added benefit, you'll extend your phone's battery life.)

Limit Bluetooth Use

Remove your Bluetooth headset as soon as you are finished with your call. Switch ears between calls so you reduce the exposure to one ear.

As an alternative, consider using a special headset called Blue Tube, which was designed to help minimize radiation exposure. Because the Blue Tube uses an air tube instead of a wire, which is found in nearly all cellphone headsets, radiation emissions are reduced.

Fight Radiation From the Inside Out

Eat lots of foods that can help support your nervous system, which is the first system in the body affected by radiation.

Foods that protect the body's cells from the potentially damaging effects of radiation are organic fruits and vegetables, organically raised red meats (e.g., lamb, beef, bison and venison), raw dairy products, egg yolks, and homemade slow-cooked bone broths.

Be sure to also include an omega-3 fatty acid supplement, which supports cell membrane integrity.

Never Wear Your Phone... Keep Your Distance

It bears repeating again and again... Do not keep your cellphone next to your body. Keep it out of your pockets; don't clip it onto your belt. Even when you aren't making a call, the phone is emitting constant radiation to connect to the nearest antenna.

And women should avoid the dangerous new habit of keeping their phones in their bras.

The fatty tissue of the breast readily absorbs the radiation from the phone, fostering tumor growth. Unfortunately, some athletic wear companies are now making bras with cellphone pockets. By all means, avoid using this clothing accessory.

Also, keep your cellphone around 12 to 15 inches away from your body when texting to reduce exposure to radiation.

Five Ways to Protect Your Family From Laptop and Tablet Radiation

Your cellphone isn't the only radiation-producing device in your home. Far from it. Although your cellphone is the most dangerous – due to the amount of time you use it and have it near you – other wireless gadgets in your life are also harmful.

And for most young children, wireless devices are a huge part of their daily activities.

Unfortunately, children are also the most vulnerable.

Children absorb more radiation than adults because their brain tissues are more absorbent, their skulls are thinner and their relative size is smaller.

As mentioned earlier, radiation from wireless devices has been declared a possible human carcinogen.

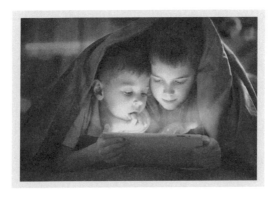

Children are at greater risk than adults when exposed to any carcinogen. Because the average time between first exposure and diagnosis of a tumor can be decades, tumors induced in children may not be diagnosed until well into adulthood.

So here are five additional critical tips and steps you must take to immediately reduce your – and your family's – radiation exposure from tablets, laptop computers and similar electronic devices.

These are easy steps. Nothing complicated here.

But they're things that most people just don't think about.

The best part is that you can start doing them immediately. There's nothing expensive to buy and no tech knowledge needed.

But make no mistake – these simple changes regarding how you use your laptop or tablet could make all the difference in the world for your health and that of your children.

Use a Hardwired Connection Instead of Wi-Fi

Who doesn't use a computer today? Nearly everyone and particularly children do...

And more and more, people are turning to laptops and tablets. Like cellphones, all computers emit radiation on many different levels.

If you're using Wi-Fi, which is often the case with laptops, placing your hands on the keyboard can cause high radiation exposure. This alone can cause a variety of adverse health effects such as extreme fatigue, agitation and numbness, tingling, weakness, and other problems in your hand or wrist – not unlike carpal tunnel syndrome.

One way to immediately cut down on the amount of radiation is to hardwire your computer. Replace your wireless installation with a hardwired Ethernet connection.

This involves simply running a network cable from your router or modem to your computer and making sure the Wi- Fi function is <u>disabled</u>. This will speed up your internet connections and reduce exposure. In the process, make sure your computer is grounded. When ungrounded, which is often the case with laptops, these devices can generate a significant amount of radiation exposure.

What I mean by grounding is that you must have your computer plugged into a three-prong outlet instead of a two-prong outlet. In a three-prong outlet, the left slot is the "neutral," the right slot is called "hot" and the slot below them is the "ground."

Use an External Keyboard and Mouse With Your Laptop

All computers, as soon as they're switched on, generate some level of radiation. Depending on how close the laptop or computer tablet is to your body, the exposure can be significant.

Studies show elevated health risks with radiation exposures as low as 2 milligauss (mG).

Unfortunately, some laptops and tablets emit significantly more than 2 mG.

The most common sources of this radiation are the motor of the hard drive inside your computer and the in-line transformer unit (all computers have some form of transformer).

By using an external keyboard, you can move your body away from all the computer components. In particular, make sure the transformer unit (often a little rectangular box in the cable) is situated at least a few feet from your body. If you have a desktop, keep the CPU at least 3 feet away from your body.

Laptops Are Not for Laps

The best way to minimize laptop radiation is to not use your laptop computer on your lap.

Studies show that, over time, using your laptop on your lap can decrease your sperm count. No man wants that. In addition, get yourself a high-quality radiation shield.

A radiation shield is a large pad that your computer sits on that deflects radiation away from your face and body. Independent tests have given high grades to some radiation shields for their effectiveness. Most shields fight multiple sources of radiation originating from your computer.

Again, do your homework.

Some manufacturers claim their shields provide 100% protection from harmful forms of radiation and reduce heat radiation.

One other thing to be aware of is computer monitor radiation. On a desktop computer, the biggest problem is often the monitor, not the CPU, primarily because the CPU sits farther away.

If you're using a desktop computer, you can use a computer radiation filter over the screen to further reduce radiation.

Use Your Computer When It's Not Plugged In

When you are using Wi-Fi, use your laptop unplugged and in battery mode as often as possible. *This alone can reduce radiation emissions and exposure by 50% to 80%.* Laptop computers are high-energy sources of radiation, so by putting them on battery power – and eliminating the high voltage that's causing the problem – you reduce your exposure to radiation output.

Most laptops, since battery life is at a premium, are set up to use less energy when they aren't plugged in. When a computer starts receiving AC power, it's often set to start running at higher speeds and thus use more energy.

Although your laptop may operate a little slower than when it is plugged into a wall... the trade-off is that you'll be doing your body a favor.

Turn Off Wi-Fi When You Don't Need It

Because we live in an increasingly wireless world, radiation will become an increasingly large danger. Most devices – desktops, laptops, tablets, etc. – now have Wi-Fi functionality. This means you're constantly being exposed to radiation.

Most computers, especially laptops, are <u>configured by default to be in Wi-Fi mode</u>. So even if you are on a hardwired Ethernet connection, your laptop is still emitting and receiving radiation.

You need to go into the settings and disable the wireless (possibly Wi-Fi and Bluetooth) functionality.

Be careful because many modems and routers are now factory configured to automatically re-enable Wi-Fi when they receive an update – this can be several times a day.

So even if you disable the Wi-Fi in the settings menu, it may be subsequently reactivated without you knowing.

Take These Steps Now

You can protect yourself from harmful radiation coming from your cellphone and computer devices.

Reducing radiation exposure doesn't have to cost you a lot of money. Start making these simple, inexpensive changes today. These strategies can be put in place by anyone.

The thing is... nobody knows just how deadly cellphone radiation will be. We won't know for perhaps another 20 or 30 years. Early evidence, though, shows we can't be complacent.

Take steps now.

Do what you can to avoid all forms of radiation. It could save your life.

We've outlined dozens upon dozens of natural cures, tips and tricks in this book that can boost health and save lives.

Now, we're not ignorant to the good that comes from modern medicine. Medicine saves countless lives every day... absolutely.

But the argument we've made here is that not all of what Big Pharma pitches will cure what ails you. And not all the system sells you is necessary.

As this book proves, you have options.

And that's certainly true when choosing the doctors who will be involved in treating, maintaining and improving your health. As Dr. Phil Roberts explains below, it's crucial to take an all-encompassing approach to your medical care in order to achieve optimal health.

The Doc Is In: A Better Approach for Optimal Health

Dr. Phil Roberts

"Fill 'er up and please check the oil and tires."

Many of us heard this phrase from the back of our parents' car as we rolled into the local gas station. While the tank was being filled, the eager attendant would check the oil and tire pressure. Often, they'd even clean the windshield. Indy pit crews came to mind as I watched them work to ensure our vehicle performed at its highest capacity.

Fast-forward half a century. Self-service pumps are now the standard. There's no one but us to make sure our vehicle is maintained at peak levels.

And if you missed Car Maintenance 101, you could find yourself on the side of the road trying to remember if your insurance policy covers roadside service. (Sadly, most folks these days are unable to properly identify a lug wrench.)

Maintaining our health is similar to the above example.

For most folks, the first few decades go by smoothly. There are no major maintenance issues... no dashboard lights to warn us of problems down the road. *Then we get older.* Here comes the widening girth... the onset of regular insomnia and anxiety... the increase of blood pressure and glucose levels...

These are all just expected parts of the aging process.

And it's up to you to recognize when there's a problem and take yourself in for a "repair." Things snowball from there. One prescription quickly follows another.

But does it have to be this way? Can't you do something about it?

Yes, you can. Allow me to pull the curtain back...

Your Treatment Options: Conventional vs. Functional

Many bad things can happen to our bodies over time. I can offer no guarantees or claims to diagnose, treat or cure any disease or condition of any kind. But I *can* share some basics.

When it comes to healthcare, the United States spends more per individual than any other country. We write the most prescriptions. And yet, in terms of healthiest nations, we're ranked *37th from the top.*

Roughly half of U.S. adults either are prediabetic or have Type 2 diabetes. Seventy-four percent have a weight problem. Fifty percent of males will get cancer sometime in their lifetime (as will 40% of females).

And 50% of adults have at least one chronic medical problem.

Last year, for the first time in decades, our life expectancy went *backward* (your children are not expected to live as long as you).

[Disclaimer: The U.S. is still one of the top countries worldwide for acute and trauma care. If you get severely injured, pray that you are in the U.S. or near a trauma unit with U.S.-trained physicians. Also note that this is not intended to offend any of my distinguished, hardworking colleagues in medicine. But it breaks my heart to see where we stand in the world ranking. My desire is to see us get back into the top 10 by 2025.]

There are two systems of medical treatment in the U.S.: the conventional path and the functional path.

As a conventional medicine physician, I was trained to treat symptoms with prescription medications ("a pill for an ill"). One prescription per decade is the norm. Your symptoms can be managed by the latest commercialized medicine that you are encouraged to request. It will be refilled at the next visit in three months.

Seeking to reverse your condition is NOT the norm. Most conventional physicians have very little – if any – training in nutraceuticals or supplements. Thus this common comment from skeptics: "Supplements provide little or no value... but they will give you expensive urine."

Yet I encourage you to go to PubMed.com and look at the number of articles on vitamin D. It's well beyond 75,000.

Many well-trained individuals think vitamin D is critically important to our bodies.

In functional medicine we seek the root cause of the illness – the etiology. Our goal is to reverse it, if possible, through the right kind of dietary foods and the correct liquids.

But the most important component is understanding the need for proper individualized vitamin, mineral and herbal supplementation. Managing stress is key too.

And so are prescription medications, if deemed essential. (I make no bones about it; prescription medications have their place and can save lives. They have saved millions of lives and will continue to be great tools.)

Bioidentical hormone replacement is also considered if your body is not producing what it did during your younger years.

Avoiding environmental toxins is wise, as is seeking to remove the heavy metal exposure.

This can dramatically reduce deadly diseases. Preventing an illness is the norm – better to prevent illness than have to cure it. (Obviously both are a win.)

But rather than choose between conventional and functional medicine, the thing you should be asking is... *Why not take the best of both?*

A Better Option

An all-encompassing approach is what I and a growing number of physicians are advocating for.

Let's not have conflict. Rather, let's share the knowledge and science of both paths.

Pride has no place here – only what is best for the patient. (That's the essence of the Hippocratic oath, after all.)

The stakes are too high. We must work together.

I believe a mix of conventional and functional treatment options are essential to maintaining optimal health as we age. There are four critical areas to address:

1. Understanding what foods and liquids to ingest and avoid

2. Taking in a customized mix of supplements based on lifestyle, genetics and familial diseases – a mix that adds back in nutrients depleted by prescription medications

3. Personalized bioidentical hormonal testing and replacement as needed

4. A plan for avoiding and removing environmental and accumulated toxins.

My goal is to help folks be like that vintage, pristine and polished 1963 red Corvette convertible you see at car shows. Despite its age, all gauges are to the "F-level" and tire pressure remains optimized.

You can just picture it roaring off into the sunset.

We are designed for excellence.

But to remain in tiptop shape... that takes work.

About the Author

Andy Snyder is the Founder of Manward Press. Featured on everything from Fox News to The Weather Channel, he's the very definition of a well-rounded man. He worked for one of the largest brokerages in the country, a firm with nearly $100 billion in assets under management. And he spent more than a decade as a researcher and investment analyst for the largest financial publisher on the planet.

But Andy's expertise extends far beyond the world of finance. He also has a background in law enforcement, is an award-winning columnist and is a best-selling author. As a guide in Alaska's remote wilds – 50 miles from the nearest telephone pole – he taught men from all walks of life how to survive and thrive by developing and relying on their own skills and relationships.

These days, when he's not tending to his 30-acre farm with his wife, two kids, three sheep, five beehives and dozen chickens, he's penning issues of his popular monthly lifestyle newsletter, *Manward Letter*, and doling out winning investment ideas to subscribers of *Manward Trader*.

Index of Miracles, Tips and Tricks